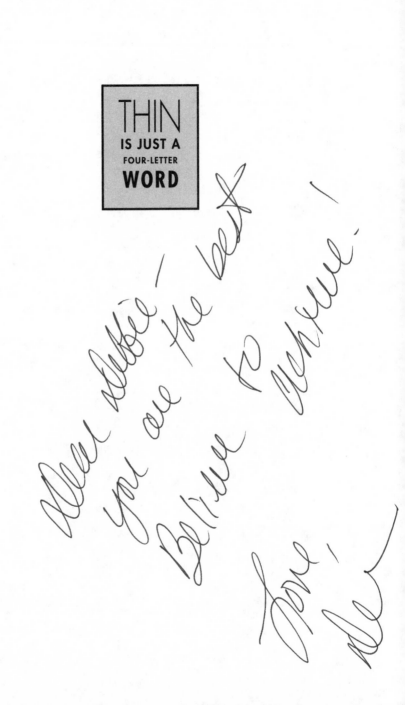

THIN
IS JUST A
FOUR-LETTER
WORD

Dear Debbie –
you are the best.
Believe to achieve.

Love,
Dan

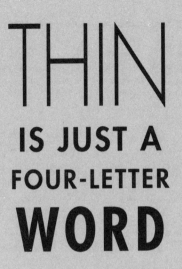

THIN
IS JUST A
FOUR-LETTER
WORD

Living Fit —
For All
Shapes and Sizes

Dee Hakala

with Michael D'Orso

LITTLE, BROWN AND COMPANY
Boston   New York   Toronto   London

First Edition

The author is grateful for permission to include the following material:

Excerpts adapted with permission from *Scan's Pulse,* Fall 1995, vol. 14, no. 4 and Winter 1996, vol. 15, no. 1, official publication of Sports, Cardiovascular, and Wellness Nutritionists (SCAN), The American Dietetic Association, Chicago, Illinois.

Excerpts on pages 89, 90, 180–183, 185–188 from *ACSM's Guidelines for Exercise Testing and Prescription.* By permission of Williams & Wilkins.

Excerpts from *Nutrition Therapy,* edited by Kathy King Helm and Bridget Klawitter. Copyright © 1995 by Helm Seminars Publishing. By permission of Helm Seminars Publishing.

"Reality Check" checklist developed by Adrienne Ressler, M.A., C.S.W., body image specialist at the Renfrew Center.

Checklists on pages 169–170 and 210–211 developed by Karin Kratina, M.A., R.D., body image specialist at the Renfrew Center.

New Face of Fitness is a registered trademark of C.H.O.I.C.E.S. VVV with De Inc.

Library of Congress Cataloging-in-Publication Data
Hakala, Dee.
    Thin is just a four-letter word : living fit — for all shapes and sizes
/ by Dee Hakala, with Michael D'Orso.
    p.   cm.
    ISBN 0-316-33911-3
    1. Weight loss.   2. Physical fitness.   I. D'Orso, Michael.
II. Title.
RM222.2.H223   1997
613.7 — dc20   96-31880

10   9   8   7   6   5   4   3   2   1

HAD

Published simultaneously in Canada
by Little, Brown & Company (Canada) Limited

Printed in the United States of America

Contents

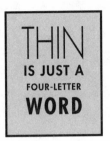

THIN
IS JUST A
FOUR-LETTER
WORD

Picture this.

It's the dead of winter in a godforsaken Gulf Coast Louisiana oil town, leaves stripped from the trees, the sky hanging low and gray and heavy, a wicked late-afternoon wind whipping across a parking lot crammed with cars.

Two women climb out of a tiny Toyota, and they're taking their sweet time about it, partly because one of them is scared absolutely witless to be here, and partly because these two women together weigh a total of close to six hundred pounds — nearly a third of a ton. Getting out of a car, getting up from a chair, just getting out of the freaking *bed* at the start of each day is enough to leave either of them gasping for breath.

The one who's shaking in her sneakers is me. I'm thirty-one years old, I've got a husband who's gone half the time cruising the Gulf of Mexico on a Coast Guard cutter,

I've got two little boys back at the house wondering what in the world Mommy's doing walking out the door wearing those big old sweat pants and T-shirt and tennis shoes — just seeing Mommy turn off the TV and get up off the couch is a shock to both of them — and I've got my only friend in the world, Ellen, squeezing out of the driver's side of that car, taking my arm and steering me toward those plate-glass doors in front of us, telling me, "Don't worry, Dee, you're gonna be fine."

Yeah, right. I'd tried this before, once, back in Milwaukee, when I was so desperate to find a friendly face that I actually hauled myself down to an aerobics studio and signed up for a class. I was pushing three hundred pounds at the time, but it wasn't my weight I was worried about so much as the fact that I was just lonely. The Coast Guard had sent us there, my husband was of course at work almost every day and plenty of nights as well, I'd just gone through my first pregnancy basically by myself, and I hadn't met a soul in our new neighborhood beyond the mailman. The people I passed when I was able to gather the energy to get out for a walk kept to themselves. I was new; I was a stranger; and I was very, very fat — not much of an invitation for an introduction.

But I was dying to meet someone, *anyone,* so I figured I'd try a class over at the club. What better place to find a friend, right?

Wrong. From the minute I walked into that workout room — actually, slunk in is more like it, I was so self-conscious and ashamed of my size — everyone there, the students and the instructor alike, edged away a little, averted their eyes, and went about the business of busting their butts to the beat of the music. I did what I could to keep up, shuffling my feet a little bit and praying for a break, hoping someone would turn around and at least say hi to me.

But no one did. Not that day, not the next, not for the year or so that I kept coming to that class. Not once did anyone in that room so much as give me the time of day. And really, who could blame them? Desperation was draped all over me, just like the folds of fat that shook every time I moved. I was a sick puppy, not just physically, but emotionally. I was wallowing in self-loathing and need-iness, crying out for a friend. And I was furious that no one was responding. That showed, too, I'm sure. Who would want to come near anyone like that?

So I quit. Screw it, I told myself. I tried, I gave it my best shot. I lost a few pounds — not nearly enough to no-tice — but I was still basically in the same place I started, still totally by myself. Sad, sorry little Dee. So I went back to the one thing I knew I could always count on, all my life, for comfort, for coping, for solace and security whenever those things weren't found anyplace else: I went back to food.

Which got me through the move down to Louisiana. Which pushed me past the magic three-hundred-pound mark for the first time in my life. Which nailed me to the sofa twelve hours a day because I had the lung capacity of a chipmunk and just about that much strength. Which made me not only unable to get up and play with my little boys, who finally learned to not even bother asking, but also trimmed my emotional fuse so short that I was snap-ping at the kids for the slightest thing, them and my husband, too. Which was putting a strain on a marriage that was already stretched to the max by the demands of our military life. Which made me realize, after a lifetime of spinning through the kaleidoscopic mental, emotional, and physical pinwheels that come with obesity, after struggling with the insidious cycle of food-focused despair and comfort that only the overweight can understand — after decades of trying to feed my soul through my stomach, I realized I was finally, literally, killing myself.

Which is why, against the objection of every cell in my body — every fat cell — I accepted my friend Ellen's Christmas gift that winter of a month's membership at a place called Gigi's, the hottest fitness club in all of Lake Charles, Louisiana. Hardbodies. Rock animals. Rooms full of high-stepping, hand-clapping spandexed men and women, all smiling through the sweat streaming down their faces.

As soon as I stepped through those doors, I wanted to go home.

But I didn't. Ellen wouldn't let me. Every bone in my body was screaming at me to get the hell out of there, that nothing was going to be different from the way it had been in Milwaukee. I was no different; in fact, I was worse. And those aerobic animals all around me, they were exactly like the ones I'd faced before, like the ones filling the rooms of every fitness center in every city in America. There was no place for somebody like me in those rooms. Who was I kidding?

But I didn't want to let Ellen down. That's what kept me there that day. And the next. And that's where this story begins, because that's where my *life* truly began, seven years ago, in the back corner of a crowded room full of strangers, where I carved out a tiny spot on that carpeted floor and finally, for the first time in my life, I took a stand.

It changed my life. Not only that, but it started me in the direction of changing hundreds of other lives, which are now becoming thousands, in fitness centers across the country, from Dallas to Des Moines, from Trenton to Topeka, from Wheeling to Waukegan, from Cleveland to Kauai — literally from one coast to the other (and farther, in the case of Hawaii), where men and women just like me are joining the program I have created, answering the call I finally heard, that fitness is not about fatness; that you don't have to be a hardbody to be healthy; that you don't have to "feel the burn" to find a home in the workout room; that the roots that are planted in that room cannot be tended just there, but must be carried outside, to be fed and watered every minute of the day; that true fitness has nothing to do with a target weight or fitting into a size 8 dress, or finally snaring that man you've been dreaming about; that fitness is a *lifestyle*, not a trip that ends with a specific goal but an ongoing goal in itself; that health and happiness begin on the inside of your body and work their way out, not vice versa; that you'll never feel good about your body until you feel good about yourself; and finally, that health is not about size or body shape, about inches or pounds, but that it is purely and simply about that organ that beats deep inside your chest.

This is the message that finally broke through my thick skull that stark Louisiana winter, and it's what has become the basis of the gospel I've been spreading ever since then. Yeah, I began in the back of that room, but baby, I did not *stay* there. No way. One thing about me — when I taste a good thing, I go for it, all the way. All my life, the one, the only, good thing I could always count on was food. But that winter, for the first time, there was something else, something that fed me as surely as any bag full of Cheetos or gallon of mint chocolate chip, and it was that knowledge, that realization, that became the foundation of the program I've developed over the past several years, a program that has drawn together hundreds of lives into a network of sweat, support, and celebration and that now has groups ranging from the YWCA of America to the Nike Corporation backing it up.

The nuts and bolts of my program are contained in this book, as well as the story of how it all came together — how *I* came together, and how you can, too. I am still obese. That's essential to understand — essential to the basis of what sets my program apart from the hundreds of workout books and videos lining the shelves of fitness sections in bookstores across America: that I and every one of my instructors are just like the students in front of us — we are *all* — every one of us — a work in progress.

I still weigh far more than I'd like to, but I weigh far less than I used to — a hundred pounds less, with thirty-five fewer inches around my waist. But more important — much more important — I am healthy, healthy enough to lead a room full of those hardbodies through a butt-kicking hour-long workout that has them drenched with the same sweat that covers me — all 220 pounds of me. I can teach twenty classes like that a week — I often have — and the beauty of it is I'm giving those students the same workout I developed with my classes of men and women with more specialized limitations — high blood pressure, rheumatoid arthritis, diabetes, and, yes, obesity.

Those were the classes I started with, the ones I created when I looked around and realized there was no place in the hallowed halls of health and fitness for people like me, for people like *us!* The outcasts. The misfits. So I made a place, starting that winter, in that little windblown town in Louisiana, starting with myself and facing the fitness industry on *my* terms rather than vice versa, rather than playing that losing game of trying to squeeze myself into the shape drummed into our heads by those Buns of Steel ads, those sculpted Soloflex infomercials, that parade of gleaming, glimmering, grinning models trotted out by Madison Avenue to show us all the way we're supposed to look. And if we don't look that way, shame on us.

Bull.

Health is about what's inside the package, not the package itself. Health is about respiration and circulation; it's about function and feelings; most of all, and there's no getting away from this, it's about the heart. Where the heart goes, the body follows. If your heart is hurting, if it's in pain, your body responds, almost always in its own wounded way. Every heart is different. Every body is different. Every life is different. Every wound is different. But we all share this basic truth — that how we deal with our hearts determines everything else about our life, from our health to our happiness to, yes, the size and shape of our bodies. Any of those things can be changed, but only by healing — literally and emotionally — the one thing that guides them all: the heart.

Let me tell you how I healed mine.

Pushed by the Dream

First things first. If you picked up this book because you want to lose weight, period, forget it. This book *is* about losing weight, but not in any way you know of — not in any way *I* knew of before I finally undertook the journey that has literally saved my life, a journey in which I've come to know, respect, embrace, and, in the truest, healthiest, most encompassing sense of the term, actually *change* a body I could hardly look at for most of my life, a body I loathed.

I'll make no bones about it; this book is partly about pain. It's about emptiness and anguish. It's about the kind of hurt that can carve holes inside all of us, holes so deep no amount of liquor or dope or sex or success or, yes, food can fill them.

It takes courage to face pain like that, to take a long, hard look at the empty places inside us, to acknowledge how those places were formed, where they are rooted, to feel the

anger, the sadness, the yearning that dwells deep down —
deep down and years back — and to turn those feelings into
forgiveness and love, first for ourselves and then for the
people around us.

It takes courage, and it takes compassion. You can't heal
something you hate. You can't help something you loathe. If
you're driven by disgust, you're headed for nothing but a
dead end. All the weight loss in the world won't help you if
you don't love what you see in the mirror when you're starting out. And if all you see is what the mirror shows you, then
you're not looking hard enough.

Vision. That's what this book is about. Seeing yourself
clearly and embracing what you see, flaws and all, understanding that there is no perfect person, there is no perfect
body, despite our culture's insistence that there is. With that
understanding constantly in mind, and with that attitude of
affection for yourself, the trip to true fitness can begin.

This *is* a book about fitness, but, again, it's not like any
fitness book you've ever read. This story is about a journey. It's
personal. It's real. It's my story, but there's a good chance at
least some of it is yours, too. I'm not here to bore you with sta-
tistics. You know the facts just as I do. You've probably lived
those facts just as I have. When it comes to health and fitness
in this country of ours today, we have a problem — a big, big
problem. You know it. I know it. But knowing we have a problem is one thing; really doing something about it is quite another. Clearly, if there's one thing we've learned by now when
it comes to doing something about our bodies, it's that this is
much more than a matter of knowledge; it's a matter of motivation. Most of us know what we need to do to really, truly
get in the kind of shape that's good for our bodies and souls.

The problem is, very few of us have figured out *how* to do it, how to stay the course and get from here to there. If someone could come up with a map of some kind, a magic map that could lead us out of the woods, out of the tangled wilderness of out-of-whack approaches to food and weight and inactivity and *hopelessness* — if someone could crack the code that keeps so many of us from doing what needs to be done in terms of taking our bodies into our own hands, that person — man, woman, whatever — could name their price.

No one knows this better than yours truly.

Seven years ago I was morbidly obese, completely deconditioned, suffering from diabetes and high blood pressure, dangerously close to death. I had struggled with weight problems ever since I was a child, problems rooted, as so many are, in the unhappiness of — and I hesitate to use this term, the buzzword that it has become — a dysfunctional family.

I don't want any part of the "victim" mentality. I like to think of myself as a fighter, a warrior, a survivor, and I *have* survived, despite a pretty heavy childhood as the daughter of a physically abusive, sexually deviant father; despite some tough teenage years, when I ran away to Florida and plunged myself into a year of drugs and alcohol and, yes, plenty of food; despite my young womanhood, when I returned home and earned a college degree, graduating with honors but finding my job search hampered by the sheer size of my body; despite the heartache of my experiences with men, again twisted and tainted by the fact that, year after year, I was growing fatter and fatter; despite my first years of marriage and motherhood, both of which saw me continue to eat my way toward a literal point of critical mass.

It was at that point, seven years ago, at the age of thirty-one, that I made the life-or-death decision to do something about my body. I'd done plenty before. I'd tried every diet on the planet. More than once I'd given the workout route a go, but nothing ever stuck. I had lost hundreds of pounds over the years, but they always came back, and more. I hated being fat, I was obsessed with my weight, aware of what I was doing to my body, guilty even as I gorged myself, driven by desperation to quick-fix solutions, always pushed by the dream of reaching a certain weight or a certain shape, fitting into a certain dress, snaring a certain man, and always finding that even if I achieved those goals, the fulfillment was fleeting, the reward was hollow, and the weight always returned.

And I couldn't figure out why.

And it kept getting worse.

And one by one, I gave up on the diets, and the exercise, and, finally, even the hope.

In other words, I had walked the same well-traveled path familiar to so many men and women, and I had wound up in the same place — overweight and devastatingly out of shape. The only difference between me and any of the 65 percent of Americans currently classified as "deconditioned" — physically unfit — was the extremity of my condition. At the point where I finally understood that my life was at stake, I was carrying well over three hundred pounds on a body that was less than five feet tall.

Naturally I felt out of place when I went with a friend to a local health club in southern Louisiana in the winter of 1989 and stepped into a room full of high-impact aerobicisers. Naturally I felt the same urge I'd always felt in a situation like that — to flee. Always, until then, I had.

But this time, for a host of reasons, not the least being that instinct for survival that had carried me that far in my life, I stayed. It was a mixture of basic stubbornness, defiance, and feistiness, fanned by a growing awareness that the goal this time was not outside my body but *inside* it, that kept me coming to those classes for weeks. Which turned into months. Which became a year.

And at the end of that year, when I had moved away from the edge of the cliff of sheer survival and was for the first time in my life reaping the inner rewards of true fitness — more energy, better moods, a steady sense of well-being and contentment — I began thinking beyond myself. I looked at the lean bodies around me and pondered the people who *weren't* in that room, the overweight and out of shape who had faced what I'd faced and, as I had done so many times before, had given up. What would it take to bring them back and keep them here? What was turning them away?

That was when I realized the answer was right in front of me. The students — most of them — and the instructors — *all* of them — were *already* fit. Lean, mean workout machines. The unfit, unfortunate few who were occasionally brave or desperate enough to venture into this circle found themselves surrounded and led by bodies shaped nothing like theirs, bodies equipped and able to do routines nowhere within reach of them, all in a setting that made few, if any, amends for the frightened, self-conscious, intimidated, physically unequipped outsider.

I knew all about the "I've been there like you" formerly fat fitness gurus, men and women who had made the journey from fat to fit, and yes, these people took the situation a step beyond what the unfit faced in those workout rooms. These figures could relate their own past to the place where their students stood at the moment — unfit and overweight. But the fact was that they and so many like them were no longer in that place. And so they were no longer one of their students. They were set apart, just as surely as any of the thousands of thong-clad hardbodies leading those high-impact classes in workout rooms across America.

And if the goal was to become *that*, to get *there*, to be like them or those instructors, then the vast majority of those students were going to wind up defeated and disillusioned, because the fact was that very few of them would ever get there. Who's to say that what's "there" for one person is "there" for another?

I thought about that. I thought about the traditional focus on body size and shape that so often displaces the realization of the rewards of sheer conditioning itself. I thought about the fact that, after a year of my own aerobic workouts there in that Louisiana studio, I was in the best shape of my life. I was still morbidly obese — more than twice the ideal weight for my height — but my cardiovascular conditioning, my muscular strength, and my flexibility had me actually in step with the students around me.

I had watched several of those students make the move to the front of the room, get their certification as instructors, and become teachers with classes of their own. And I thought, why not me? Why not become one of the insiders, then turn around and offer the outsiders — the unfit who truly did *not* fit — a place, a program, and an *instructor* who was one of them?

It was as if I'd found religion, and I went after it like the Holy Grail, getting my certification, gathering a precious few first students — some overweight, others suffering from rheumatoid arthritis, a couple with diabetes, all for one reason or another outcasts and casualties on the standard fitness landscape — and watching that class swell until I had to create another, and another, until soon my students outnumbered the hardbodies enrolled in the regular classes, many of whom, curious about what exactly was the appeal of what I offered, tried my class themselves and became converts, getting all the workout they wanted and more — getting a sense of connection and support that extended beyond the classroom, that went beyond simply pounds and inches and reached into issues of self-esteem, body image, personal relationships, family issues, and so much else relating to true health, well-being, and happiness.

Mine is — again, hold your breath for a buzzword — a holistic approach to fitness, with an essential ingredient in my program being the requirement that my instructors reach out and respond to each student on the *student's* terms, discovering and defining their particular conditions and limitations and beginning there, rather than requiring the student to meet or adapt to the standards set by the instructor.

And that is where my story — and my program — hits a gear and strikes a chord unlike any other. Because what I did — and what I and the instructors I've trained are continuing to do at this very moment, as my program has begun branching out to cities across the country — is something different from anything offered before in the crowded arena of health and fitness. It's human. It's empathetic. It's honest. It's demanding. It's responsive. It's effective. It's connective. And it's hitting a target audience that until now has remained largely untouched, so much so that the industry itself is sitting up and taking note.

Two years ago, a panel of national fitness experts chose my program from among dozens across the country as the winner of the Nike Corporation's inaugural "Fitness Innovation Award."

But let me make clear right here that this book is not meant to sell you shoes or sell you on my program. The only thing I want to sell you on is yourself and your health and moving your body! I'd love nothing more than to see your face in one of my classes. But if I don't, what I do want is for each and every person who picks up this book to come away from it with the motivation, knowledge, and determination to take their body and life into their own loving hands, to get up and get moving on the path to true fitness, a path that has no end. Do it alone. Do it with others. Do it with me. But *do* it.

This book will show you how. It is the story of my life, a story of loss and lostness, of desperation and discovery, and finally of the light that can shine within any of us once we find our way onto the path of true inner and outer, physical and emotional, muscle and soul *fitness*.

I'm pretty sure you'll find some of yourself or someone you love in my story. I hope it can help you find understanding and compassion for that person, and that that understanding can point the way toward the path of true health and happiness, a fantastic, unbelievably and amazingly bountiful path that has no end.

See if this story doesn't turn you toward it.

2

Two Different Lives

So where do I begin? Where do any of us begin but with our childhoods, with our families, where the seeds of our selves are most deeply planted. I know that's where mine were sown, in central Michigan, in the late '50s and early '60s, in a household that, on the face of it, was Ozzie-and-Harriet ideal but in fact was a frightening minefield of sudden, terrifying explosions, bursts of rage from my father that would detonate without warning, then disappear just as quickly, like the summer squalls out on nearby Lake Huron.

I was actually born in Sacramento, in 1958, the first of my parents' three kids, each of us named by my mother, who was on a *D* trip at the time. There was me, Dee; then came my sister, Darcie; then my brother, Darrin. My Dad's name was Leland, but everyone called him Skip. Skip and Sharon, those were my parents, a standard '50s couple,

Dad away at work every day while Mom stayed home and raised the children.

My memories begin in Michigan, where we moved when I was four. My dad had started his own janitorial business in the Flint area, and that's where we lived, in a split-level, semisuburban home with a boat in the driveway and a convertible in the garage. Most days my dad was gone before I was up. My mom would usher us out to play or, as time went by, send us off to school, then turn to the house, mainly the kitchen, where cakes and cookies were constantly coming out of the oven. There were three square meals a day on the dining room table, meat and potatoes every night, a prayer before digging in — my mom was a staunch Baptist — all of it picture perfect, except for the fact that my father was an alcoholic, a nasty drunk with a nastier temper.

He'd be gone for days at a time sometimes — his job was like that, with whole office buildings to clean and crews to manage — and then he'd come home like a hurricane. My mom would say something, *anything*, and that would set him off. All hell would break loose. He'd start flinging furniture around, breaking a lamp or a picture frame, knocking doors down.

The only time he ever hit me was one my mother had to tell me about because I was much too young to remember it myself. I was ten months old, to be exact, and my dad came home from work one day totally exhausted, completely wired. He'd had a few drinks, and at that moment he was apparently just not into being a parent. I was crying, as babies will, and my mother couldn't get me to stop. She could see my father getting more and more pissed off at my fussing, and she started getting scared. But she couldn't get me to quit. Finally, all of a sudden, my father grabbed me and threw me — *threw* me! — across the room. I hit the railing of my crib and landed on the floor like a broken doll. My mom was petrified. I wasn't breathing. She didn't know whether to take me to the hospital or what. She was basically in shock. And my father stormed out of the room.

It wasn't until years later that I learned this story from my mom. By the time she told it to me, she had finally been forced to face the dark side of this man she had married, a side she denied during the seventeen years they were together, a darkness rooted, I now know, in my father's own troubled childhood. Like me, his seeds were sown early on, something I haven't truly understood until fairly recently. Seeing our parents not as some larger-than-life, mythological figures but simply as human beings — flawed human beings — takes a long, long time, but it's essential, I've learned, to understand them that way in order to understand ourselves. We may not forgive them for the wrongs they did us, wittingly or unwittingly, when we were little children. We may not even be able to bring ourselves to love them. But we can understand them.

I understand now that both my dad's parents were alcoholics. One of them, my grandfather, eventually cleaned his act up, but not before he'd totally screwed up his son. The one incident I know of, which is enough in itself to make me want to forgive my dad for every horrible thing he's ever done, happened when he was just a boy.

My aunt Marie told me this story, that my dad came home one day with a little puppy he'd found. He was so excited, just as you'd expect a six-year-old to be. When my grandpa got home that night from work and saw this puppy, he wanted to know who gave my dad permission, who told him he could have this dog? And he didn't wait for an answer. He took the dog and my dad both out to the backyard and made my father watch while he shot the little animal through the head. Then he made my father watch while this tiny puppy ran around the yard until it dropped dead.

How sick is that? How can I blame my dad for anything he became, no matter how awful it was?

And it was awful. By the time I was in grade school, our family had settled into a routine of nightmarish scenes behind closed doors, coupled with a superficial surface of suburban serenity. It was as if we were living two different lives. We went to church three days a week, I was in the popular group at school, I hung out with the cool dudes, I made great grades, dressed in the nicest clothes, had tons of friends. It was always, "Hey, let's go over to Dee's house," and my mom — the chocolate-chip-cookie mom — would always have great snacks waiting for us on the kitchen table, fresh out of the oven. She was always ready to take all of us — eight of us, ten of us, whatever — skating. And she'd throw these hellacious birthday parties. Great birthday parties.

But I knew even then that it was all her way of making up for the times that my old man had torn the crap out of the house, turned the dinner table over or something like that, put us all through pure unadulterated hell, and didn't blink an eye the next morning when we'd all head down to the church, a good Baptist family, happy and smiling and wearing our Sunday best. Never mind that my father had been drinking in the basement of that same church on Friday night, when he went to clean it. Come Sunday morning we were right there in those pews, singing hymns and praising the Lord.

Two different lives, that's how I grew up. That's how we all grew up, my siblings and I, and naturally we reached out for whatever anchor we could find, a grip, something we could turn to for the assurance of normalcy in the face of my father's relentless rage. One place we found it was in the food on our table.

More than half of all the terrifying things I went through in my childhood happened at the dinner table, because that was the one time you could always count on my dad's being around — dinnertime. I can remember countless instances where we would be sitting around the table, Darrin and Darcie and my mom and me, and someone — maybe one of them, maybe my mother, maybe me — would inevitably say or do something that would set my father off, and he'd suddenly explode, just go completely ballistic. It might be Darrin telling a joke too loudly, or Darcie saying something my dad didn't like, or my mother asking him something about money or wondering where he'd been for the past two days — I don't think that if you're married and you want to know where your husband has been for two days, it's wrong to ask — and he'd blast off, just go crazy. He'd purposely go over and grab something that my mother had sculpted — she was an artistic person, very good with ceramics — and he'd smash it to pieces. Or he'd pull the phone out of the wall. Or he'd pick up his plate and fling it. Or he'd pick up the whole *table*.

And what did we do? Were we allowed to go run and hide, or cry, or even give a hint that every cell in our bodies was exploding with fright? Did we have permission to have *our* emotions and show them? No. We had to stay at the dinner table, pretend nothing had happened, and *finish . . . our . . . meal.* We were scared to death to move.

It didn't matter that our heads were spinning inside from the scene that had just happened, that the whole world seemed to be coming apart, that later that night all three of us kids would wind up downstairs in my basement bedroom hiding under the bed, whimpering but keeping it quiet so he wouldn't hear us, while he went on another tirade, maybe pulling out a gun and threatening to shoot my grandmother for bringing my mother into the world — I'll never forget that one. Never mind any of that. No matter what, we were supposed to pretend that everything was fine, and that meant cleaning the plate, every bite. Keep it normal. Keep a grip. Do that for five, or ten, or how many years and tell me you're not going to have a little problem with food.

Physical abuse can be evidenced by bruises and scrapes, but it's the scars on the soul left behind long after the wounds of skin and bone are healed that are truly devastating. It's those wounds of the heart and soul that we treat in ways we don't even realize. We're just kids when we begin developing coping mechanisms. We do what we need to survive, and we don't even think about it. Years later we might figure it out, but not then. How could we? We're just little children when the dye is cast, when we start turning in directions that affect the entire course of our lives. The direction I turned in was food. For my brother and sister it was something else. We all cope in our own way, develop our own mechanisms to deal with the turmoil that invades us. What are *your* mechanisms? Think about it. How do *you* cope?

Of course I had no clue at that time that food might be a problem. On the contrary, it was a blessing, a haven, a comfort I could count on. Believe me, when you're in a situation like that, you cling to the happy stuff wherever you can find it, whatever it is. Food. Friends. Whatever good stuff you can find.

Unfortunately, this good stuff made me fat. By sixth grade, I was beginning to hear the taunts and teasing. "Chubby Checker" some of the kids called me. My girl-friends were beginning to get their first boyfriends. I'd see some of them strolling home from school holding hands, sneaking kisses. I walked home alone. I compensated in the classroom, always at the top of my group, and I had a great personality, was always surrounded by a circle of friends. But when it came to boys, it never went further than friends.

I remember a boy named Fred Buchanan coming up to me in seventh grade. "You've got a really pretty face, Dee," he said. "If you lost thirty pounds, I'd go out with you." How many times did I hear *that* during my teenage years?

My father was a big man. Not tall, but big. Short and chunky. It was my mother who always had a weight prob-lem, and by junior high school, I started dieting with her all the time, trying this and that. My mother went from be-ing pretty badly overweight down to a normal size dozens of times, and now I began joining her, bouncing back and forth between losing a little weight, then turning around and eating those chocolate chip cookies till the cows came home. That old rubber-band diet syndrome — the starve-then-gorge cycle — I got to know it early.

We tried every diet in America, my mom and me. The grapefruit diet, the water diet, the protein diet, and let's not forget the pee-on-the-little-stick-and-see-if-it-turns-purple diet. If that stick was purple, we were losing! If it didn't, we weren't. I remember that time in my life when the sheer ecstasy of my entire day was based on the shade of purple of that stick. It was like, "Well, Mom, we're having a PURPLE DAY!" My whole sense of self-esteem was based on the color of that little sliver of wood.

By high school, I was the classic firstborn child, the achiever. I was in the National Honor Society, secretary of my class, a member of the school's chorale group, traveling around the state to sing in public. I was overweight, and attracting boys remained a problem, but finally, when I was fifteen, I met a guy named Mike Weaver. We went to the same church. Weekends Mike worked for my dad, helping clean the church. We started dating, Mike and me, first with a group of other kids, then by ourselves, and pretty soon we were a couple. For a year and a half we went steady. I had never been so happy. Then suddenly, with no explanation, Mike stopped coming around, stopped calling. It was a week before I was able to track him down.

"What's going on?" I asked him.

He didn't say anything. He wouldn't even look at me.

"Come on," I said. "What's going *on*?"

Finally he looked at me.

"Your dad hit on me."

"He *hit* you?" I said. I couldn't believe it. I mean, everything was still bouncing off the walls with my family at home, but my world outside was pretty okay, pretty normal. I couldn't believe this, that my dad would actually hit somebody outside our family the way he sometimes hit us.

"Dee," Mike said, "wake the hell *up*."

I'd never heard Mike use a single swear word before.

"I didn't say your dad hit me," he went on. "I said he hit *on* me. He made a *pass* at me. Your dad is *queer*."

I felt as though I was going to throw up. I had to close my eyes, my head was spinning so badly. I couldn't say a word, I couldn't think a thought. I just stood there, mute, numb, literally blown away, completely scoured out inside, from head to toe.

I hardly remember what happened the next couple of days. No details. It was as if I was in shock. I guess I *was* in shock. I don't know where Mike went, where I went. All I know is, once my mother found out, she finally made the move she hadn't been able to bring herself to make until then. Her religious beliefs had always held her back from even considering such a thing as divorce. She'd be damned in the eyes of God if she even thought about divorce, that's what she believed. But when she got wind of what Mike had told me, she went to our minister for some counseling. He told her that what my father had done was basically considered adultery, that that's the way God saw it, and therefore she would not go to hell if she left this man.

So she did. She told my father to move out, which he did, but not before adding another memorable scene to the nightmare side of my childhood. As angry as he often was, my dad has always turned positively radiant when it came to my achievements in school. He bought me books, tons of books, from the time I could first read, and he'd brag to whoever would listen about his bright daughter, his honor roll girl. By the time I was in high school, I had shelves and shelves of books, from Dr. Seuss to Shakespeare. Encyclopedias, atlases, everything.

Well, the day my dad moved out, he pulled all those books down, every one of them, hauled them out to the backyard, piled them up, and set them on fire. And he made us watch, just the way his old man had made him watch that puppy die back when he was a little boy.

Then he left, moved into an apartment of his own. And believe it or not, I missed him. That's the way kids are, so desperate for the love of their parents that they'll do anything, forgive anything, to keep that connection. Even after all he'd done, this man was still my father. No matter what he did, he couldn't make me hate him. I didn't care about school anymore — the bottom dropped out on my grades and I quit the chorale. I didn't care how much I weighed — I was shoveling food into myself as fast and as much as I could. But I still loved my daddy, still pedaled my bike over to his apartment almost every day, just to see him. Until one afternoon he answered the door and blew away any shred of normalcy I might still have felt about his life or mine.

I'd come to get the keys to my dad's old Chevy station wagon, which he'd told me I could have. When he opened the door, I thought I was at the wrong house. I was looking at someone I had never seen before. This was my father, but he was wearing high heels. He had on a dress, a black dress, with black hose. And a wig. And nails. And makeup. And he had this voice, this feminine-pitched voice.

"So what do you think of your old man now?" he said.

It felt like land mines going off inside me. I flipped. I backed away, reeling, left my bike lying in the driveway, and drove off, my stomach churning, blinking back the tears even while I pushed the accelerator to the floor.

I wound up at a friend's house that night, drinking myself into a stupor — my father had taught me how to drink by then, sometimes sharing a bottle of peppermint schnapps with me when I'd go with him to help with a cleaning job. I overdosed on PCP that night as well — my first experience with drugs. When I came to, I'd been to the hospital, had my stomach pumped, and was back at my friend's house, lying in a tear-soaked bed.

That was it. As soon as they let me out, I threw a suitcase of clothes and my puppy into that station wagon. It was a piece-of-junk Chevy, it drank oil faster than gas, but it could get me where I wanted to go, and where I wanted to go was as far south as I could, driving until the road ran out and all that was left was ocean.

Florida, that's where I was headed. Welcome to the real world, that was my logic. Your dad's screwed. Your mom's screwed. Your life's screwed. So it's time to leave.

Sixteen years old, and I was out of there. Gone. Alone.

Magic Man

I spent a year in Florida, moving in with an aunt who lived in a small house within walking distance of Daytona Beach, right on Highway A1A. I was basically a teenage runaway, working odd jobs for pocket cash, drinking quite a bit, smoking a lot of marijuana and doing mushrooms, anything to obliterate my memories of the mess I'd left behind in Michigan.

I was doing all I could to climb into the present moment, living right *now*, running away from the past, and paying no mind to the future. I was anesthetizing myself, something you can do for only so long before there are long-term prices to pay. Thank God, I only lived that way for a year, long enough to put some distance between where I'd been and wherever it was I was going. And long enough to put on some serious weight.

Think about it. Drinking like that can't help but make

you fatter. You go to a bar or a concert, drink like a fool, wind up puking your guts out for the next day and a half; then you're hung over and dehydrated, your body's crying out for fluids, healthy fluids, and all you want to do is eat. So I was into that cycle pretty much the whole time I was down there. By the time I left at the end of that year, the one good thing I had to show for my stay in the Sunshine State was a killer tan.

I came back to Michigan in the autumn of 1974, back to my mom, who was remarried by then, living on a farm with her husband, way out in the country, with cows, corn, the whole 4-H deal. It's not hard to imagine how I stood out in that setting, the bad chick who had left home. I had this long blond hair down to there, skin dark as chocolate, and I was *big* — about 150 pounds. I remember somebody in my stepfather's family saying, "Boy, she looks like a round brown ball."

Mom was still into making these huge meals, even huger than when she was married to my dad. Cows and cream and homemade butter. Milk straight from the cow — none of that homogenized stuff. Meat and potatoes and gravy every night. Food, food, food, food, *food*. I was back now to the rhythm I'd left before, the good girl doing what was expected of her — chores around the farm, my schoolwork. But school was no longer the source of comfort and happiness it had been before I ran away. This was just a little country town, not that many kids, so everything you did or were — or *didn't* do or weren't — really stood out. Or at least that's how it felt.

I went to the junior prom by myself. Nobody invited me to go with them. I bought this halter dress that was gathered in at the waist, then hung straight down — a pretty good coverup for my weight, which was by then pushing 160. My mother sewed an extra sash around the waist to help cover things up a little more, and away I went.

Walking into the gym-turned-prom paradise, I thought to myself, What a joke! Did I think Mister Magic Prince Man was going to suddenly appear and invite me to dance the night away with him? Well, one can always hope.

Of course the fact was that that fantasy remained just that. Tell me if you've been through this one: sitting or standing through a night like this, trying not to look as alone as you actually are, as you actually feel, trying to put on that happy face, ever so slickly acting like you're having the time of your life, a dream evening.

In reality, I couldn't wait until my mom came to pick me up. Not one dance all night. That was my junior prom.

That was a tough two years for me. I wanted so badly to be a part of everything, to belong, like any teenager. But I didn't. I didn't know these kids, and I'd been living a different life from them; they'd been going along doing the high school thing while I was off traveling, on the road, smoking dope, doing the wild thing. So I turned to eating and studying. Those became the two focuses of my life, and I threw myself into each of them with equal enthusiasm — especially the food.

The funny thing is that some of that overeating came from the fact that I was actually more active than I'd ever been before. My farm chores had me up every morning at the crack of dawn, putting milkers on the cows, getting them into their stalls. This was *work*, and in a weird way I used that as a license to indulge myself even more at mealtime. It was as if that little bit of activity justified absolute scarfing at the dinner table. Hey, I told myself, I'm working out now, I sweated a little bit today, and I earned this. I've noticed this little phenomenon many times in my life, and I'm pretty sure you can probably recognize it, too. Those little mind games we play with ourselves to justify the things we do. Nudge that door of rationalization just a sliver, and it may as well be wide open.

Let me slip in a little subnote on this particular topic, if I may. Once I became a fitness professional and began studying the body, especially people who are overweight, one of the first things I learned is that activity drains the body of necessary fluids — dehydration. Simple enough. But what makes it a bit more complicated is the fact that that activity also drains the body of something called glycogen, which is what glucose becomes once the body breaks it down and stores it.

Here's the kicker. When a person who has been inactive — especially an overweight person who has been inactive — first begins moving their body and getting active, they might be thirsty, but even more than that, they find that their *hunger* has increased. Or at least they feel hungry — even more hungry than they'd be if they hadn't worked out.

It's happened to me so many times. I finish working out, it's an hour or so after I'm done, I've cooled down, it's getting close to mealtime, and I'm like, WOW, am I hungry! I mean, I'm famished. And I know I've just worked out, and I feel good about that, and I think, Hey, I deserve to feed this hunger. I've earned it. And so I gorge myself, not realizing that what my body is translating as hunger is actually a need for FLUIDS.

H_2O.

Water.

Hydration.

Nothing will stem that inordinate post-workout "hunger" and give the body what it actually needs like a tall, ten-ounce glass (or two) of cool, clear water.

And if you're still hungry? Well, you may be, but then you've got to assess what kind of hungry it is, because the fact is that it's probably get-a-glass-of-water-and-a-piece-of-fruit hungry. Or have-a-glass-of-juice-and-a-bagel hungry. In any case, I can guarantee you it's probably not an eight-ounce-steak-three-helpings-of-mashed-potatoes-four-ladles-of-gravy-and-a-small-portion-of-green-beans hungry!

Oh yes, those green beans. Toss a couple of them on the plate and your meal is suddenly healthy, right? That little piece of parsley on the edge of the dish makes the meal well rounded. Aren't we proud of ourselves? Got the veggie thing covered there, uh-huh.

Man, the hoops we can jump through in our heads.

Believe me, no one out there is more mentally acrobatic about these things than yours truly. Thinking ourselves through our problems, and sometimes thinking ourselves completely out of reality . . . hey, it's just another way of coping. And really, coping — and recognizing the root of that coping behavior — is what this story, and *yours*, is all about.

By the time I graduated from high school in the spring of 1976, I was coming out of adolescence and aching both in my heart and my body to explore relationships with men. Unfortunately, *because* of my body, those relationships would become a tangled source of heartache and shame that would continue for years to come.

Sex. I began groping my way into that territory once I started college, and for several reasons, not the least being my self-consciousness about my size, it was terrible. Ninety percent of the time, if I came to the point where I wanted to go to bed with a man and the opportunity was there, and the situation was right, and the man was someone I cared for and he seemingly cared for me, I wouldn't do it, because of my body. Those occasional times when I did actually sleep with someone, I'd do little things like wear a skirt that I could remove without taking off my top, so the man wouldn't see any more of my body than necessary. Or I'd medicate myself, have so many drinks that I'd lose my inhibitions enough not to worry about what he thought of my body.

I was ashamed. Embarrassed. And how did I respond to that shame, how did I make myself feel better? I ate, which made me even larger, bringing me more shame, and more food. Creamy. Crunchy. Yummy.

I was confused, almost blind, when it came to my dependence on food, my use of it as a crutch, and I was just as blind about the pursuit of intimacy. Rather than finding fulfillment within myself, I searched for it through a mate, and I searched for a mate by treating my body as a mere means to that end. Almost every time that I made an effort to lose weight in my life, the motivating factor was a man. I wanted to be with someone, I wanted someone to care about me. Of course that's not the right reason to do anything. Of course I had to care about *myself*. But I didn't know that then.

And so I got trapped into that spiraling cycle of food being the focus no matter which way I was going, losing weight or putting it on. When I was lonely, food was my comfort, my consolation. It made me feel better. It made me happy. Then, when I wanted to go after a man, I'd try to diet and exercise and maybe it would work or maybe it wouldn't. I love to bike. I'm talking about an outdoor, take-it-on-the-road, breeze-in-your-face bike. It's so different from a treadmill, or an indoor stationary bike, or any machine in a room with four walls. Outdoors, with my Walkman strapped on, my music in my ears, the scenery passing by while I roll along — there's never been anything quite like that for me.

There certainly was never anything like it in an aerobics room full of people. That way lay fear, humiliation, self-consciousness, heartache, intimidation. You name it. I imagine that's part of what drove me to solitary-activity pursuits at an early age — going for walks by myself or riding my bike. Get me away from others' eyes. That and get me outdoors, which I have always loved. Maybe it comes from that midwestern upbringing, but I really do draw a vibe from nature, from the earth itself, from the trees rustling around me, the sun warming my skin, the wind blowing through my hair. Hey, maybe it sounds corny, but it's true. And it's good. And it's real.

Grooving on my bike, taking in the green, the hills, just *going,* just feeling so alive. Can I express how fantastic that feels?

But did I know back then the value of this activity as

an end in itself? Did I understand that this might be part of the mind-set that could take both my body and my soul where they needed to go? No. It was something I did that felt good, but meanwhile I was chasing desperately after something else — specifically, after the companionship of a man — and I wound up like a gerbil running inside one of those wheels, getting nowhere. I'd twist the purpose of activity, aim my workouts at losing weight, pervert the process of eating by doing the diet thing, lose some weight, and no matter the outcome, always wind up alone again, back in the same familiar place. Either I didn't get the man or it didn't last if I did, and I'd say, Screw it, and I'd go back to what I knew, to what was always there for me. And what did I know? I knew I was happy when I ate.

I hadn't truly been in love, hadn't been able to get that far with a relationship, since my high school boyfriend Mike, the boy my father had shocked out of my life. I'd been able to do pretty well for myself in terms of independence, earning a student grant to get myself into a small school not far from home, a place called Northwestern Michigan College, and finding a part-time job to help pay my bills — for my car, my apartment. I was dying to meet Mr. Right, and finally, near the end of my sophomore year, I met a man who loved me for who — and what — I was.

His name was Terry Gilmer. We ran into each other at an outdoor concert and it just really clicked. We felt so comfortable with each other. He was a big guy, about six three, and pretty hefty himself. He'd gone through losing quite a bit of weight, and so it was almost like he related to me. He'd never been with a woman, or not many, because he used to be really big, so this was the first time in his life that a woman paid attention to *him*, was attracted to him, loved him the way he was. And he felt the same way about me. We stayed together for almost two years, among the happiest two years of my life.

For the first time in my life I lost weight without trying. The reasons, though not apparent at the time, are so obvious now. I had a roof over my head, I wasn't worried about paying my bills, I was doing great in school, and I was living with a good man who loved me. I felt so good about me, so safe and secure, more than I'd ever felt in my life. I didn't *need* food as much anymore. There was nothing desperate about my life anymore. That hole inside me was filled with something else now, something more substantial than food — and a whole lot less fattening.

Not that I wasn't still way overweight, and not that I didn't want to do something about it. I didn't like being fat. I never had. I was always, constantly, trying to lose weight even as my lifestyle was piling it on. But this time, for the first time, I had a foundation of security to help me work at it. I *had* a man, so the motivation to lose weight was coming from within myself, to please myself, not someone else. I was far from understanding what true fitness was about and allowing that to be my motivation, not just how I looked but how I felt as well. It would be years and years before I would begin to develop a whole, healthy, loving relationship with my self and my body. Meanwhile I had a lot to learn, including the lesson I got through my time with Terry.

It started out great. I felt a willpower I'd never experienced before, based on the security of the things I knew I had no matter what — most of all, my boyfriend. I weighed about 160 when I decided to join Weight Watchers. And it worked. I stayed the course and dropped about forty pounds — within about ten of my target weight of 110. I could actually fit into a pair of painter's pants with a 29 waist. I was feeling fantastic. I mean, men were looking at me, really paying attention. That was a pretty incredible feeling, an amazing sensation. I'd never had that before.

And then you know what happened?

Terry dumped me, that's what happened.

He started getting insecure that summer. He noticed men starting to notice me, and began getting jittery about losing me. So he put the power trip on, began telling me I didn't need to do any more of this healthy-eating stuff. "Come on, Dee," he'd say, "let's go out and have pizza tonight." And I'd go, because that's what he wanted.

And the weight started coming back. Between the end of that summer, when I'd dropped to 120, and that Christmas, I gained sixty pounds. Sixty. That put me at twenty pounds *heavier* than when I'd begun Weight Watchers. Winters have always been a hard time for me in terms of activity because it's hard for me to get outside. It has been ever since I was twelve years old. I suffered a wicked case of frostbite that year up in Michigan. Our church group went on a ski / toboggan outing one weekend, and I was having such a blast, I didn't notice that my feet had turned numb inside my soaking wet socks and boots. By the time I got home that night, they had actually begun turning black. It was nasty. My folks rushed me to the hospital and I turned out okay, but the doctor told me I'd never be able to have my feet get cold again. And I haven't. I don't even risk it.

So I tend to be an indoor person in winter, and for the longest time — too long — being indoors meant no activity. It also meant, that winter of '77, at the urging of Terry, lots of eating. So my weight ballooned, and in the meantime Terry was closing in on graduating from nursing school. He was approaching a crossroads in his own life, and as that time approached, he began pulling away from me. God knows the web of reasons, the complexity of things he was going through. My size hadn't mattered to him when we first got together, but after he'd seen me thin and healthier, it seemed as though my size *did* matter. And this time around I wasn't just big. I was *huge*.

Did Terry dump me because I was fat? We never really went there. But I'm sure that was part of it. And it's important to point out that it wasn't just my size, but how I wore it, what it did to my self-esteem, how I felt about myself, which was absolutely, 100 percent crappy. When you walk around loathing yourself, people can feel it. They move away. Who wants to be around that? How can anyone expect somebody else to care about you when you don't care about yourself?

I know now that this wasn't about Terry. It was about me. It was *always* about me.

I didn't realize then that it doesn't matter how many legs you have, how many arms you have, how tall you are, how small you are, what color you are, what color your hair is, what color your eyes are, or whether you look like Jane Fonda. When you feel good about yourself, when you're trying to take care of *you*, when you're happy with just the mere effort of taking steps in the right direction, in the healthy direction, of caring for yourself and your body, it radiates from you. Other people see it. Other people feel it. You walk into a room and they know it. Their response to you is a direct result of what you're giving out. It's simply an attitude. Your attitude about yourself.

By that Christmas of 1977, my attitude about myself was lower than low. Then Terry dumped me. And I couldn't believe it. I'd helped him get *his* confidence and self-esteem up just the way he'd helped me with mine. I'd made him safe and secure and strong just as he'd made me — or I *thought* he'd made me. He finally got strong enough, as it turned out, to leave me.

And so there I was, still screwed up more than I realized, still measuring myself by someone else, still putting my self-esteem in another person's hands rather than my own. Still alone.

It's pretty ironic, when you think about it, that the first time in my life that I lost weight without a man being the motivation, I lost the man.

It broke my heart.

A Person My Size

By the summer of 1979, after Terry had left me the winter before, my waist size had swelled back from a 29 to a 36. I was despondent, depressed. If it were not for my two dogs, Suki and Thor, mother and son, white German shepherds, the absolute loves of my life, I would have had nothing. And when my landlord told me I had to get rid of the animals or move out, I started packing. It was the summer before my final year of college. I had no job at the time, my bank account was on the thin side, to say the least, and so, rather than hunt for another apartment, I decided to take the tent I normally used for camping and try it out as a full-time home, nothing but me and my pets living out in the forest.

I wound up on an island, actually, part of a state park. The government offered permits that allowed long-term camping, so that's what I did, set up a home for myself and my dogs there in the woods. It was a rugged life, a bare-bones existence — and it turned out to be the best medicine I could have found for both body and soul.

I was collecting unemployment at the time — about thirty bucks a week. I could only afford so much for food, and what I bought had to keep without refrigeration. My refrigerator was a Styrofoam cooler and ice — that's what I lived out of.

I couldn't buy much in the way of fruit or vegetables because they'd go bad. The same with meat, plus I couldn't afford that. So basically I lived on popcorn and potatoes — lots and lots of fried potatoes, which I had to walk two and a half miles to the nearest store to buy. When it was time to cook, I had to gather firewood and kindling. And there were the dogs to take care of, walking and running with them all the time.

At first it was hell. I cried a lot. But I was determined to do this. I was more alone than I'd ever been in my life, completely alone, but after a while that became beautiful. I'd sit out in this one field almost every morning, get out there just before the sun would rise, and the grass and trees would be wet with dew, and the sun would come up and everything would suddenly sparkle, just burst into glittering light. Deer would appear and not even notice I was there. I had never felt so at one with my soul, writing down my thoughts, poems, soaked in the magic of the moment. I can't tell you how enchanting those mornings were. Amazing. Really magical. I told myself I would never forget those mornings — this "soul time," if you will — and I never have. To this day, I can put myself back in that place, just like that.

It wasn't long before the rhythm of my days, contrary to what might seem at first like hardship and deprivation — which is what it did seem like at first to me — began to become a comfort, then a joy. I'd rise each morning and hike along upstream behind my tent to a spot where the stream met a larger creek and formed a fairly deep swimming hole. The water was cold as ice, but the river bottom was soft, smooth sand. No rocks whatsoever. It was as if God made this little oasis so Dee could bathe. It was so cool.

I didn't disturb anything. I never even broke a twig. I'd carefully hang my clothes on a nearby tree branch, then I'd dip myself into the water, then I'd climb back out to soap myself, and then, before getting back in the water, I'd wipe off the soap with a towel — I didn't want to put any of those chemicals into that crystal-clear, clean-enough-to-drink water.

By the time I finished each morning's bath and got back to the campsite, it was time to gather wood. That in itself was a time-consuming — and though I didn't notice at the time, a calorie-consuming — adventure. Practically the entire heart of my day was built around wood — hunting for it, finding it, trimming it with a handsaw, hauling it back to my campsite, often over a distance of half a mile or more, then sorting it into stacks of different sizes, from twigs and kindling all the way up to logs.

Those neat stacks of wood reflected the orderliness of my entire campsite. I guess I got that neatness bug from my mother. A place for everything and everything in its place. That's the way it was in our house when I was a kid, that's the way it is in my house today, and that's the way it was in that campsite. It may have been just a little tent and my belongings, my cookware, my wood supply, and the pile of empty cans I collected each day scavenging along the roadside and in the woods — that aluminum brought me a couple of bucks a week when I went into town to buy food — but all of those items were arranged as neatly as an army recruit keeps his bunk in boot camp.

The days actually began to fly by, believe it or not. Factor in my daily romps with the dogs, and evening came pretty quickly, which meant bedtime. I had no lighting to speak of, and I didn't need it. Since it was summer, I had daylight till about 9:30, and by that time I was ready to turn in. I was beat — that delicious feeling of a body tired from an honest day's work.

By the end of that summer, I was not only more content than I'd ever been by myself, but I had also burned off enough calories and fat to be in the best shape of my life. By no means was I thin — though I did drop about forty pounds, down to about 150 — but I was in tremendous condition. Call it a deprivation diet, or a *survival* diet, along with forced exercise. It's not a routine I would recommend, but it worked wonders for me that summer.

Unfortunately, in terms of my health, I had to move back into town that fall to finish my last year of school. The exercise that I had had no choice but to get that summer went out the window, I returned to a lifestyle of virtual inactivity, eating on-the-run, easy-to-grab prepackaged and fast food, and finding that the size of my body had an enormous impact on the career I was planning to enter.

My major was marketing and merchandising, and my goal was to get into retail clothes merchandising, to be a buyer in the fashion industry. I'd always dressed extremely well, no matter how much I weighed, no matter what conditions I was living in. I might have been overweight, but I was *never* a slob.

That's something I learned early from my mother, I guess, something that always helped keep me fitting in. Looking nice, the art of dressing yourself, the strategy of putting together outfits that hide your obesity — these are all skills that a fat person develops. You'll never see me in shorts, for example. The same with horizontal stripes or floral prints. Even if I were thin, those patterns would not be flattering to me because I'm short and my face is round. Add a large body to that, and you've got a recipe for a visual disaster.

I learned to put together outfits that were not tightly fitted, that didn't adhere to my shape but that hung in an attractive manner, that accented the elongation of my body rather than its width. I always had a knack for dressing myself well, and I was just as good with other people. My friends used to ask me to help them shop for clothes or put an outfit together. Colorwise and in terms of separate pieces, it's a matter of assessing a person, of being able to step back and see what works with each individual's features, and I guess there's a little bit of natural creativity thrown in there, too.

In any event, I had that talent. I knew how to make myself look nice, even being overweight, and I wanted to make a career out of doing it with others.

But I never got that chance. Both during school — through work-study programs and internships — and after graduation, I found myself turned away whenever I sought a position with a clothing company. It didn't matter that I had all the academic credentials, that I had the sales skills, or that I had this great sense of clothes and clothing. It was a visibility thing. Nobody would hire me, because of my size, and who could blame them? Who would want somebody trying to sell clothes they couldn't even fit into?

So I wound up working in the one industry where a person my size might look — and feel — at home: the food business. I became a manager at a McDonald's, then at a Howard Johnson's, then at an upscale department store in Evansville, Indiana, where I was put in charge of the gourmet food section. Wines, coffees, cheeses, Godiva chocolates — we carried it all, and I enjoyed it all. That, and access to the store's restaurant, where I ate well, really well.

I got that job with my sister's help — she had moved to Evansville a couple of years earlier — and I lost that job because of my sister, who had scars of her own that she was still dealing with. While my legacy from our childhood had become an eating disorder, while I was trying to fill the hole in my soul with food, it turned out that my sister was doing it with other substances. I was stunned, to say the least, when a bad-check incident on her part drew me into a no-win situation with the department store management. Basically, I was given a choice to either press charges against Darcie and keep my job or take a hike. Press charges? *As if*. This was my *sister* we were talking about. So I packed up and moved, back to the one person who would always take me in, no matter what — Mom.

Nice shot for the self-esteem, huh? There I was, twenty-six years old, with a college degree, back home in Michigan, living with my mother, weighing more than I

ever had in my life and working down at the Cherryland
Mall as an assistant manager in the House of Flavors
restaurant.

Naturally I was continuing to eat, continuing to put on
the pounds — I was back up to about 190, which is where
I'd been before my summer in the woods. And like too
many women in my situation — closing in on thirty with
no man in my life — I was feeling more and more desperate to find a mate.

What I did find were a lot of men who were overweight
themselves, nice guys who would approach me for a date,
and my reaction to them would be the same repulsion I
faced day in and day out in my own life. Hard to believe,
but it's true, not just for me but for many overweight
women I've talked to. Their feelings are constantly bruised,
their hearts are constantly broken by people who reject
them because of their size, and yet they often find themselves turning around and responding the same way when
confronted with an overweight man.

I remember one guy in particular who wanted to become friends with me — a good guy — and I rejected him
because I knew he wanted to be more than friends and I
wasn't attracted to him that way in the least. It was the
weight thing, pure and simple. I imagined what he'd look
like with his clothes off, and that really turned me off. It
disgusted me.

Now you tell *me*, how hypocritical is that?

The best I can do is plead ignorance. So much ignorance back then. About myself. About what matters in life.
About the lessons that are learned when you finally know
how to listen to your heart and listen to your body.

I was still years away from learning those lessons, years away from identifying and beginning to resolve the dizzying swirl of issues that caused and were caused by my obesity.

Little did I know, those issues were about to multiply beyond my worst nightmares, with marriage, motherhood, and the life of a military wife.

5

Down the Tubes

His name was Keith Hakala. He was twenty-two, four years younger than I was, and he was a "Coastie" — a Coast Guard sailor. He'd come from a midwestern family, like me, and I was attracted to him the minute I met him, at a party a friend had to drag me to because I was so self-conscious about my size. I actually stayed outside in the car at first, and I might have stayed there all night if this friendly blond guy hadn't strolled out and coaxed me in. He actually seemed to think I was cute, talked to me all that night, then called me back a few days later, just like he said he would. He seemed down-to-earth, honest, and, best of all, he didn't seem to care about my weight.

Keith was used to overweight people. He was relatively slim, but everyone else in his family — four siblings and both parents — was heavy. He accepted that in them, and he accepted it in me, accepted me for who I was.

I've got to admit I was feeling pretty desperate at that time. I'd been seeing a guy just before Keith, and he'd just given me the big 10-4. He was actually a great guy. Charlie Sampson was his name. Straight out of the pages of a biker magazine. Long hair, a long beard, he could've been one of those dudes in ZZ Top. He rode a huge Harley Super-glide and looked tough as nails but was actually one of the gentlest, sweetest men I ever knew. Just the kindest soul. But like so many men, all he had to hear was the mere mention of the words "marriage" and "commitment" and he was out of there. I love you, Dee, he told me, but marriage? Unh-unh. I don't think so.

There was nothing ugly about the way Charlie and I parted ways, but still it was that abandonment thing kicking in again. That, plus my age and my bottom-of-the-pit self-esteem, put me in a position of being pretty hungry for affection. Keith showed me that affection. Plus, he had the most *normal* family I'd ever met, galaxies away from the one I'd grown up in. This was a man I respected. A good man. A kind man. A caring person, someone I could see would be a great father. I fell in love with everything about him, with the way he seemed to live his life, with his integrity, his solidity, his family — the whole package. Was there any way I would even think of saying no when he asked me to marry him? And it wasn't the skinny Dee he was asking. It was big Dee, the heavy Dee. It didn't matter to him what size I was. I was *Dee*, and that's what he loved.

We met in April 1984. That October we got married. Two months later Keith was assigned to a base in Milwaukee, and I found myself completely alone, in an apartment without furniture — the military movers had lost it — in the dead of winter. Keith's training kept him away for days at a time. I didn't know a soul and didn't have much opportunity to meet anyone, and so, for the first time in my life, I joined a fitness club — not to get in shape but simply to find a friend.

It was a little aerobics studio, in a redbrick building downtown, not far from where I lived, just a couple of minutes' bus ride. The room itself was on the second floor, which was a workout in itself, just climbing those steps. I was pushing two hundred pounds by then, the most I'd ever carried, and let me tell you, carrying myself up those stairs was not easy.

Well, it was clear from the first day that this club had the persona of the "Itsy Bitsy Teenie Weenie Yellow Polkadot Bikini" all over it. Picture the person who would actually *wear* a bikini like that, and you've got an idea of the kinds of women I saw shooting up and down those stairs. Some of the outfits I saw in that place had about as much material in them as a bikini. I can look at that kind of getup now and ask myself, What's the point, but back then, all I remember feeling was complete and utter awe. Looking at this room filled with these gorgeous female bodies was like standing in a museum and looking at artwork. And coveting it.

Suffice it to say I was not wearing anything close to a bikini. Quite the contrary, I was wearing as many clothes as I could possibly pile on. Huge sweatpants, gray of course. And this massive purple (size 4X) long-sleeved, thick, heavy shirt. Every time I put it on, I'd sit down and stretch the edges of it over my knees so it'd sag down and hang as loosely as possible around my hips and my butt. Anybody who's ever been big knows that trick by heart.

My feeling was that the more covered up I was, the more loosely my clothes hung on me, the more protected I was — literally insulated from stares and judgment. No one would see the bulges and the rolls and the fat folded over — the stuff I saw when I dared to look in a mirror. Somehow, I felt, I wouldn't look as big with all this stuff on. Of course the fact was I *did* look big. But that wasn't the point. These are the little things you do with your mind to try to save some face. I'm sure it didn't mean a damn thing to anyone else, but this was my reality in my head.

As for the reality in the heads of the women around me, it was unmistakable. From the first day I showed up until nearly a year later, when I finally quit, almost every one of them looked at me as though I were from another planet — if they could bring themselves to look at me at all. Some of them acted as if I were contagious, as if I represented their worst nightmare, the very thing they were there to get away from. It was as if my mere presence might somehow be catching. Here I was, trying to find a friend, and instead I was scorned and rejected, treated like some kind of leper. Who needs that?

So finally, after about ten months, I went back home, sequestered myself in the apartment, and attacked the refrigerator with renewed vigor — until I found out I was pregnant.

I actually lost weight during that first pregnancy, which was pretty incredible, because the body creates a lot of new fat cells during that time and that usually compounds the problems for a woman who is already overweight. Typically, an obese woman will gain a really significant amount of weight during a pregnancy, and most times she'll wind up keeping most of it.

But that didn't happen to me. I had a job at the time at a pet store, and I rode my bike to work, which was good for my health, especially since I was beginning to have high blood pressure problems. My doctor was happy about the bike-riding, but that didn't explain my weight loss. What did explain it — at least part of it — was a drastic shift in my eating habits, a weird, unexplainable taste I suddenly developed for healthy foods. It wasn't a conscious effort on my part; it was biological. As soon as I became pregnant, I could no longer stomach the foods I had always craved, the things I normally devoured as a matter of course. Pizza and chips made me sick. The mere sight of sugar buns or doughnuts made me ill. But salads, they went down great. Fruits and vegetables, I couldn't get enough of them. It was as if my body took over and made me eat what was good for it.

Our first son, Zach, was born in 1986. Less than two years after that, I was pregnant again. By then, Keith was away for weeks at a time, tending buoys on the Great Lakes, which left me alone to deal with a pregnancy that was nothing like the first one.

This time around I hated salads, I hated apples, I hated oranges. All I wanted was ice cream and buns and doughnuts. I didn't care how unhealthy it was; everything else made me sick to my stomach. I could see my body practically ballooning before my eyes, but I didn't care. My justification — and I knew the whole time that this was pure bullcrap — was I'm pregnant anyway, I'm going to get fat anyway, so to hell with watching what I eat.

I not only gained an incredible amount of weight during that pregnancy, but I also developed gestational diabetes. My blood sugar level was off the scale, my blood pressure was sky high, and when my doctor performed an amniocentesis a month before I was due, he decided to deliver the baby then and there rather than wait any longer. My body was too unfit, too unsafe, to carry the child any longer.

I was a medical nightmare. I knew it. So I told my doctor, Dr. Karnes, a lovely man, I'd decided not to have any more children. I told him I wanted a tubal ligation. "You're going to have my guts open on the table anyway," I said, "so just go in and do the snip-and-cut. Please. I'm done."

I was only thirty years old, a fact Dr. Karnes emphasized when he answered me. And his answer was stunning.

"Now I want to say this to you, Dee," he said. "Normally at your age I would make you wait, because you just never know. Right now I know that's how you feel, but you might not feel that way a few years from now. And if you did, we'd talk about it and make a decision then.

"That's what I would *normally* recommend," he continued. "But to be honest with you, in your current state of health, in your current condition, if you were to stay like this — and you haven't indicated to me that you intend to do anything to change it — becoming pregnant again would be very dangerous, a very high risk situation."

In other words, he was saying he'd never agree to do this with a normal person, but because of the fact that I was such a physical nightmare, he was going to go ahead and grant my wish.

That was rough.

And so my second son, Jeremy, was born, a healthy, happy baby. And Dr. Karnes granted my wish — the tubal ligation was performed.

Tubal is a pretty apt term to describe the course my physical and emotional condition took over the next year — it went right down the tubes. Soon after Jeremy was born, Keith was transferred to the other end of the continent, from Michigan down to Louisiana — Lake Charles, Louisiana, a thousand miles from anyone I knew and a world away from any place I'd ever lived.

This was oil country, Gulf Coast oil country, smack-dab halfway between Houston and New Orleans. The next town over was called Sulphur, which tells you just about everything you need to know about this section of Louisiana. "Petrochemical complexes," which is a fancy way of saying oil refineries, are everywhere you turn, popping up among the palm trees and moss-hung oaks like big metal mushrooms.

Hot, humid, swampy — the air itself made me feel I'd landed on another planet. You'd step outside and try to breathe and it was like being underwater. The weekend we got there, there was a hurricane. I'd never been in a hurricane in my life.

Then there were the mosquitoes, and the ants, *fire* ants. It seemed they were everywhere. Every time I went outside with the kids, we'd get stung by these ants from hell. Which were nothing compared to the roaches. The house we rented was full of them, the biggest roaches I'd ever seen, so big they'd come up and salute you and shake your hand. I'll never forget, not long after we got there, I had a nightmare that an army of these roaches came and chewed off a chunk of land, and I lost my family because they were floating away on this piece of ground that had been bitten off by these insects.

It was awful.

Keith, as always, was gone most of the time, on drug patrol down in the Caribbean or tending buoys in the Gulf, and again I knew no one. And I didn't feel I was worth knowing. People could hardly look at me without turning the other way. It was getting to the point where I could hardly look at myself. Any self-esteem I had had just about completely vanished. My education, schoolwork, the academic success — that all seemed another life away. My career, my professional skills, my savvy — that was far behind me. When I looked in the mirror, I saw a failure, a worthless, fat person who had spent her married years giving up her own life and living through her husband's career, drawing any sense of adventure or of being alive from him.

I felt like a complete and utter zero, and I looked like it, too, at least through the eyes I was using at that time. All the negative stuff of my life, both my past and my present, I had come to own, to believe, to accept everything I didn't like about myself and my life and identify myself with it. I was bad. I was a loser. And my body image simply fed that disgust. The only time I ever used a mirror was to put makeup on. I certainly wasn't there to look at my body. In fact, the whole time I'd be in front of that mirror working on my face, the rest of me would be screaming, "Hurry up! Get done what you've got to get done so you can get away from this piece of glass."

Mirror, mirror, on the wall, who's the fattest of them all?

That would be me.

That was my mental attitude. That was the role I had accepted for myself. That was the place I'd put myself in. It had nothing to do with other people and what they did or didn't think. It was what *I* thought. It was *my* judgment. Okay, I told myself almost every day, you're basically a low-life nightmare.

Total surrender. Guilty as charged. And the sentence? Confinement to my house, my tiny, air-conditioned fortress with its well-stocked refrigerator.

How can I describe how much food meant to me at that point in my life? It didn't talk back. It never let me down. It made me feel creamy, and it made me feel loved. I could crunch with it, I could sing with it, I could wallow in it. I could have it melt in my mouth. I could sit there and do it all, lose myself in the whole box, the whole bag, the whole bucket.

And I did. I completely let go. McDonald's french fries, Lay's potato chips, Hamburger Helper — I could eat an entire box of Hamburger Helper by myself, easy. Cheddar Cheese, Lasagna, Beef Noodle — every flavor. One box is supposed to feed how many, six? I'd eat it all myself. And remember, that's with a pound of meat.

Kraft macaroni and cheese, the same thing. And ice cream, oh how I loved ice cream. Mint chocolate chip. Rocky Road. I could eat a whole half gallon. Not right out of the box. A bowl at a time is the way I'd do it. But it'd be one bowl right after the other, so it might as well have been straight from the box.

Food. At that point, I thought it was all I had. I don't think I'd ever felt quite that way before. Every other time

I'd dealt with a food crisis in my life, it had involved trying to get a man. Gotta get a guy, gotta get thin, and then the rebound effect when it didn't work out. That's the way food had been twisted for me in the past. But this time it wasn't about a man. This time there was no yo-yoing involved. This time it was a one-way trip, period.

As bad as my habits had ever been, now they were worse. There was no holding back. My eating had become compulsive, a sickness, and I knew it. Still I kept at it, devising strategies familiar to so many millions who have traveled this road, playing games with myself and my family to hide what was happening.

Making dinner, I'd taste everything, telling myself that was part of the preparation process. A spoonful of this, a spoonful of that, another spoonful, one right after the other, pretty soon you've eaten an entire meal before you've even sat down at the table.

Then there were the kids' plates. I'd pile those up with food, and of course they'd only eat a little bit. Then I'd finish it off, clean their plates. Hey, people are starving in Africa, right? Can't throw good food away now, can we?

Finally, it started getting really sick. Lying and hiding and sneaking. I'd have a party, and I'd put just a few little dinky bits and pieces of food on my plate like everybody else, but then I'd duck into the kitchen and hide around a corner and stuff my face while no one was looking.

Or I'd wake up in the middle of the night, get out of bed real quietly so I wouldn't wake Keith, sneak down to the kitchen and pull out a half gallon of ice cream, eat half of that and put the rest back in the fridge. Keith would pull it out the next day to have a bowl and he'd say, "Geez, didn't we just buy this? It's already half gone!" And I'd say, "Oh yeah, Zach had a bowl last night."

I mean is that some sick stuff or what, using your own children to cover up your lies?

I've done some counseling work in women's shelters and crisis centers, and I've dealt with more than my share of alcoholics and drug addicts, and I can say that there was not much difference in my behavior when it came to food and the behaviors I saw among the women with drinking and drug problems. I knew what it felt like to be so crazed for a "fix" that you'd actually consider robbing a bank to get the money if need be. You're that utterly desperate. You're not thinking straight anymore. You're numb to everything but the feeling you get from that "drug" — which in my case was food. You're so unhappy that those precious few minutes when you're high on crack, or stone drunk, or in a cheap motel room with some sex-for-pay — name your addiction — are worth whatever you're doing to yourself and to everyone else involved in your life. How you're doing harm is irrelevant. All that matters, all that exists in your head at the moment, is getting that fix. And you'll do anything to get it.

That's what addiction feels like. And the fix itself? It's almost like a trance. You're not even really there when you're doing it. It was as if my eyes had rolled back in my head and I was just hand-to-mouthing it in. It was like pounding a punching bag — the unleashed emotion, the fury of it, the intensity, the vindictiveness and resentment and rage, the lashing out. Except instead of a fist pounding a bag, it was the food pushing into my mouth.

Now wouldn't it be more constructive to find an actual

punching bag and go and pound on that thing? Of course it would, and that's what I do now. I take my inner stuff, whatever's gnawing at me, and find an outlet that's good for me, that's healthy. I call a close friend and hook up to do something. I get up and move, literally shift my body, shake things up. I go work out. There are so many choices besides my "drug."

Think about *your* drug, whatever it is. Think about how you slide into that state, give yourself over to the fix, aren't even really there when you're doing it because you aren't in charge, the "drug" is, and when it's over, when you "wake up," you're like, Omigod, what did I do? But you do it again, and again, and again.

That was me, stuffed, full to bursting, slumped on the sofa after a binge-eating session, feeling physically ill, a tiny voice in the back of my brain saying, This has got to stop, this can never happen again, just look at yourself.

But it would happen again. And it did. Again and again.

I could see I was nearing a breaking point, and so could Keith, who until then had never commented on or complained about my physical condition. Now even he was noticing. I had become so big that I had absolutely no desire to have sex anymore. We'd been married for years, and Keith had always been comfortable with my body, as big as it was, which made me comfortable about physical intimacy. I was never ashamed, never felt like I had anything to hide with him. But now I didn't even want to take my clothes off in front of my husband.

He started to make comments, too. Nothing ugly, just a mention here and there like, Gee, you've gotten big. Or he'd see how I couldn't even bend over and tie my shoes anymore, how I never went out of the house, how I was in this perpetual funk, this angry, irritable mood, and he'd say, If you're so miserable, why don't you do something about it?

Of course that's easy for the other person to say, and it's the last thing someone in my condition wants to hear. It never sounds like helping, even though it's meant to be. What it sounds like is blaming, finger-pointing, and that's how it's heard. Believe me, that's how it's heard.

By the winter of 1989, I weighed — hold your breath — well over three hundred pounds, almost three times the ideal body weight for my height. I was suffering every minute of the day, barely able to move or even breathe, yet always able to summon the strength to reach for the refrigerator door. I was thirty-one years old, and my life had hit rock bottom. I had, both literally and figuratively, reached a point of critical mass. I was dying, and I didn't know what to do about it. I was sick and tired of being sick and tired. I felt I had so much to offer — as a mom, as a wife, as a *person* — but I was trapped in this miserable shell. I loathed what I'd become, this culmination of a lifetime of hurts and learned behaviors and coping and survival mechanisms. My whole life had been about filling a void, making something that hurt feel better, and what I was doing just created more hurt and a bigger void, everything just heaping higher and higher.

I needed to find a way out, but it couldn't come from Keith. I can't explain why, but that just doesn't work. Your husband, your wife, maybe they're just too close, too involved in too many ways — whatever the reason, they're rarely the one who can help pull a person out of the situation I was in.

You've got to have help, there's no way to do it yourself, and that help has to come in the form of a person you trust, someone you respect, someone you believe in, somebody who can step into that void that's always been there and can take your hand and make you believe they're not going to let go, they're not going to abandon you and leave you hanging the way you've been left before, somebody who can say, I'm not going to give you any more excuses, and you can hear those words without blame, without shame, and you can start taking the first steps to turn yourself around. You need someone to hold your hand who really cares, be it a man or a woman.

In other words, you need a friend.

That winter of 1989, I met that friend, a woman named Ellen Langley. And finally, for real, my life began to change.

Call Me Blind

That winter of 1989 I had truly hit rock bottom, the pits. I'd been miserable for a long, long time, but now my life was literally on the line. I needed to do something, but I had no idea what. Another diet was out of the question. Was there a diet on the planet I hadn't tried?

I felt I'd given the fitness route a go as well, at clubs like the one I'd tried back in Milwaukee. All that ever made me was bitter. I'd feel people were turning their backs on me, shutting the door in my face, and that would send me away angry, even more committed to staying the way I was. My reaction would be, This is the way I am, the way I've spent most of my life, and you should accept me this way, and if you don't, you're a lousy person.

Basically I would wallow in a mixture of anger and self-pity. Take me as I am or screw you — that was my attitude, which is the stance of so many of these "Fat Acceptance" groups that have sprung up in the past few years. I under-stand and agree with the no blame—no shame part of these groups' philosophies, the acceptance of a person for who that person is, no matter the size or shape. That's ab-solutely the place to start, but that's just the *start*. To say to people, "Hey, I'm overweight, I'm out of shape, and if you've got a problem with that, that's *your* problem," might be true to an extent, but it misses the other half of the equation, which is that it's *my* problem, too, because if I'm overweight and out of shape and I don't do anything about it, or at least try to do something about it, it's probably go-ing to kill me.

I can accept myself and love myself, fat and all, and I should. I need to. But that doesn't mean I'm supposed to embrace the fact that I'm fat and stay that way, because the fact is, if I'm fat and I'm not doing anything about it in the way of exercising and eating, then I'm not healthy. And if I'm not healthy, the bottom line is that I'm not going to be happy.

So no, simply sitting back and saying, Take me the way I am or get lost, is not the answer, at least not for me, or for anyone who has a choice about changing their physical con-dition.

The problem was, I didn't *have* an answer. I was wary of weight-loss groups, with their focus on food itself rather than on the source of the hunger that craves it. Diets, food plans, the hundreds of programs fixated on what and how much we eat, all seemed to simply feed the cycle of weight loss and weight gain. I knew that much. I knew I needed to get at the root of my hunger to really change anything.

I thought about therapy, but I couldn't afford it. I picked

up a self-help book here and there, but they didn't take. I was not the type of person who could cure herself. Some people are like that, they can do it solo, and more power to them. But that's not me. I needed the company and support of other people. And I guess that's why, when I saw a notice for a meeting of a local chapter of Overeaters Anonymous that winter, I jotted down the date and time, and I went.

It wasn't easy going in the first place, all by myself. And it wasn't easy doing what was demanded of everyone there, which was to be brutally honest with yourself, to really assess who and what you were and to start looking at how you got there.

I mean, I'd survived for thirty-one years by forgetting where I'd been, by focusing on the present, by taking whatever came at me and dealing with it, saying, Okay, this is what I've got to handle right now, today, in order to get to tomorrow. I didn't spend time looking back. Why in the hell would I want to look back at my past? I was trying to get *past* my past. My mother used to say it over and over again: "This too shall pass." I had spent my life saying those words to myself, repeating them like a chant. *This too shall pass.*

Now, with this group, which was based on the same twelve-step process as Alcoholics Anonymous, I finally began lifting my eyes from where I was or where I wanted to be and started looking back at where I had been. It was hard — actually, it was excruciating — but it helped me take the first steps out of that cycle of self-soothing and self-loathing through which I had been spinning my entire life.

I know this sounds unbearably New Age, but the fact

is, I finally was able to let myself feel my feelings instead of pushing them down and covering them with food, the way I'd been conditioned back when I was a kid, when I was taught to act as if everything was okay even if it wasn't.

I'd always prided myself on being strong and clung to the fact that I was strong, I was a survivor. Deep inside, though, I was actually petrified to let myself feel sad, because if I did, it might never stop, that sadness. It might just swallow me up, there'd be so much of it.

Let me say something about this sort of sadness, about understanding what's behind that word. It's a sadness that starts out small, like a single tear, but it grows, because it has to, and soon it's a river, a constant flood of heaviness and hurt, consuming you, swallowing you, wrapping around you until it becomes all that you know. The ache of this sadness, this hopelessness, this nothingness — it's perpetual. It doesn't go away. You wake up with it in the morning, and you go to bed with it at night, and yes, tomorrow is another day, but the hell of it is, it's no different than today.

The clinical term, of course, is depression. We know this. But knowing something intellectually and actually living with it are two different things. I have known this kind of sadness. I have felt it, and as painful as it is, the feeling itself is the first step out of it. Not masking it. Not numbing it. Not evading or avoiding it, but feeling it without shame or blame. It's so important to understand this, that it's *okay* to feel our sadness because that feeling, that acknowledgment, that openness to the pain is the first step on the road out of it, the road that sets us free. As the saying goes, there's no way around it but through it.

That's what I was able to finally begin to start doing, to face my feelings without fear, to say to myself, If I'm sad, I'm going to go ahead and cry. And if I'm happy, I'm going to soar so high you're not going to be able to keep my feet on the planet. And I started to see that I didn't have to earn my happiness or worthiness by making great grades, or being a great businessperson, or having a great personality and lots of friends; I could be happy with the simple fact that I'm *me*, that I exist, that I'm on this earth and alive right now.

It took quite some time to arrive at that revelation. Before getting there, I had to confront my feelings about my dad. I'd done a good job over the years of tucking those feelings away, putting all that horror behind me — or so I thought. But it wasn't behind me. In fact, it was present every minute of the day, and it was at the root of so much of my behavior, including, of course, the eating.

I came to realize, first of all, that my feelings for my father, which I'd thought were hatred because of all that he'd done, and disgust because of all that he was, were actually the pain of love — love kicked in the teeth by abandonment.

He had left me. I realized that *that* was what had been gnawing at my heart all those years. It wasn't his homosexuality that bothered me, though I had always assumed that was a big problem. It was the reason my mother split up with him. It seemed so important. But I realized it wasn't. I realized I didn't care if he slept with elephants, he was my dad and I loved him. And because I loved him so much, it hurt me incredibly that he could push me away, leave me behind, abandon me. I didn't hate him. I *missed* him.

I realized that that was a big part of the hole inside me, the hole I'd been filling with food for so many years. I was killing myself by trying to kill the pain and sadness I felt about my dad by overeating. Now I realized that the pain and prejudice I'd come to know so well because of my size was the same sort of pain and prejudice my dad had to have suffered from because of his sexuality, because he wasn't straight.

I could forgive him for that now. I could forgive him as well for the anger and rage I'd grown up with. God only knows what he was dealing with inside himself. What was harder to forgive was the fact that, in the end, he had left me. And by recognizing that fact, I realized for the first time in my life how my eating was connected to my pain. For the first time, I understood that this wasn't about food. It was about feelings, and specifically it was about the incredible web of feelings rooted in my childhood.

Finally, the loose ends of my life were beginning to link up, including the revelation that I didn't have to prove myself worthy of love to anyone in this universe, that I — as well as every other person on this planet — am precious and unique and lovely by virtue of the very fact that I exist.

This idea hit me like a lightning bolt when I was going through the OA process of writing an inventory of people I had wronged in my life. I was talking with my OA sponsor, a woman I came to have incredible respect for, and somehow we got on the subject of the great grades I'd made in school and how that was just about the last time I'd felt good about myself. She stopped me and said, "Dee, don't you know that your self-worth has nothing to do with your brains, or what you know, or what you do? You have worth,

Dee, because God made you. Even if you weren't smart, you would be worthwhile because you are YOU, the only Dee in the entire world!"

Maybe it sounds corny, but I can tell you those words hit me at that moment like a bolt from the sky. They pierced right into my heart, and they've stayed there. I'll never forget those words. That was the day I began believing in myself. That was the day my positive affirmations began — the process of writing down the things you want to feel about yourself and repeating them over and over until you do feel them, and then continuing to repeat them after that because they are true.

I have worth because I exist. Can I tell you how that sentence has become ingrained in my heart?

I love my Dad. Can I tell you how that sentence liberated me, freeing me to feel both sadness and joy about myself and the world around me?

Once I realized I didn't have to cover up my sadness and pretend it wasn't there, once I was able to, yes, feel my feelings, food finally began fading as the focus of my life. Happiness, sadness, pleasure, pain, all my problems — none of it was about food anymore.

Here is where I began taking my first baby steps on my new lifelong journey to health and my new face of fitness. Food had been my tool, my coping tool, my happy pill, my lonely pill, my everything. Now I was learning that I wasn't wrong for developing a tool; I was a survivor, and that tool had kept me sane, to a certain extent.

I have no doubt that my whole compulsive thing with food was simply my continual attempt to fill the void, to soften the sadness. Think about it. Where do eating disorders in general come from? They come from attitudes and misconceptions about what is acceptable, and those things collide with a person's own feelings of inadequacy, their lack of control of other things in their life. The result is acts of self-sabotage, bingeing and purging, starving oneself and then turning around and eating until the cows come home, and then eating some more.

It's a way of punishing oneself. It's a way of trying to feel or be "acceptable." It's a way of finding comfort. Pick your favorite eating disorder, and I can bet you I've hit the nail on the head regardless of what you actually picked. It's that "all or nothing" syndrome. No happy mediums allowed in today's world. I look in the mirror and I decide I disgust myself, then I heap on the images that society bombards us with, add in the pressure to belong, to be "in" rather than "out," to be acceptable to my parents, to my peers, to friends, to strangers . . . to mySELF. And the pressure grows, and the cycle spins, and the pressure grows some more, and on, and on, and on.

"Be the best."

"Be the thinnest."

"Be the sexiest."

"Be the smartest."

It's enough to make a body and brain go crazy. But "going crazy" is not acceptable!

So what do we do? We find secretive ways to cope, to control, to fight back in whatever way works for the moment. And one moment leads to another. And this little eating thing becomes compulsive overeating. It becomes bulimia. Or anorexia.

Hellohhhhh! Is anybody out there?

As I began to put it together, to sift through my past and sort out what had caused what, I realized for the first time what effect exercise had had on my life — not formal, organized, in-the-gym exercise, but the simple routines of a physically active day-to-day life.

I thought back to the times in my life when I'd been relatively thin without being on some crash diet, and I realized that every one of those times was when I was forced by the situation I was living in to be active, to simply *move*: when I didn't have a car so I had to ride my bike to work; when I lived in the woods by myself; when I had two dogs I had to walk and run with every day. And I thought to myself, Aha! Though this had been a food thing all my life, maybe I could make this an activity thing, since activity had always made me feel so good. Maybe this *should* be an activity thing. What a concept!

Maybe this wasn't about size, either, I thought. Maybe it was about how I *felt*, physically and emotionally. And if activity made me feel better, then that's why I should do it. What if I traded out some of the "not so great" coping mechanisms and brought in some new, healthier ones? I could feel good and accomplish a lot of great things in one stroke. What if I reprioritized why I was going to use activity in my life, not spend so much time concentrating on the size issue but on how I felt after I sweated. What about how I feel after a hot bubble bath? How I feel after a good heart-to-heart talk with a friend? How I feel when I listen to my favorite music?

Feeling whole. Feeling serene. Feeling accepted and embraced and loved by others and by myself, because I chose to do something good to help take care of myself, and nothing more. No standards to be met. No goals to be achieved. No conditions to be satisfied, other than being, purely and simply, ME.

Activity and exercise, what I eat and how much I eat — I could see these things becoming part of my life now, not because of how they would make me look, but because of how they would make me feel. This had nothing to do with losing weight, at least not directly, though that would naturally come along with it. It had to do with how I would feel, inside, where it counts, not outside, which had been the focus all my life.

Call me blind, but I'd never thought about this before.

It was one thing, however, to realize the truth, and quite another to do something about it. If I hadn't met Ellen, I probably would never have done anything about it.

Ellen Langley was a lab technician with one of the oil companies in Lake Charles. She was older than I was by about ten years. Like me, she was overweight, nearly as large as I was. But Ellen had a calmness and self-assurance about her that I had never known. That fascinated me, drew me to her. And Ellen was drawn to me, maybe because I was so many things she was not, both good and bad. It became kind of a big sister–little sister relationship, with you-know-who as the kid.

We became fast friends, Ellen and I, and finally I had found what I needed. Finally I had met a mentor. Without Ellen, I might have gotten no further than *thinking* about what I needed to do with my body. Thanks to Ellen, I took the first steps toward actually *doing* something, beginning that winter of 1989, with a Christmas present from Ellen: a month's membership at the hottest fitness club in Lake Charles, a place called Gigi's.

I would never have gone near that place if Ellen hadn't come with me. And I was amazed when we walked into this room filled wall to wall with perfect bodies and Ellen strode right in as if she owned the place. I was speechless, looking over at her, big just like me, acting right at home, chatting with everybody, seeming so comfortable, as though she belonged. I definitely did not feel that way. All these people in their thongs and spandex, and me in my sweat pants and the biggest purple shirt I could find and my high-topped tennis shoes. I felt so self-conscious.

Once the workout began, things got worse. My self-consciousness was displaced by utter despair. The warm-up alone damn near killed me. I was pretty much dying after three minutes. Everyone had their arms up over their heads, stretching, and I couldn't lift mine past my shoulders. They all bent to touch their toes, and I couldn't even *see* my toes, much less touch them.

Then the warm-up ended and the actual exercise routine began, and I just could not do it. It's not that I didn't want to do it. I just couldn't. Two or three minutes of faking it, tapping my toes or whatever, and I had to stop, go over and sit on the bike. Which made me feel like even more of a freak than I was already feeling. And I thought to myself, "Why am I subjecting myself to this pure and unadulterated hell?"

But this time I had an answer. I looked over at Ellen, and I put my mind on everything we'd been talking about, everything *I'd* been talking about, and I told myself, No, you are not going to quit. You're going to stay here if it kills you.

And it felt like it would. It felt that way for a long time. Ellen would show up in her "Really Red" sports car, and part of me would be excited to see her, to have a friend, to have something to do other than sit in the house and eat, and part of me would dread seeing her pull into the drive. It was like that old double-edged sword, my feelings running on and off, happy and frightened, up and down. Let's face it, the way I was raised, it was always like that. I'd had a lifetime of either singing in the church choir or hiding under the bed scared to death. Drastic-land. Opposite extremes. I knew them so well.

What kept me going during those first six months was Ellen's presence and her attitude, those small amounts of hope. Because at last I was at least trying and not just sitting on the couch in my misfit, pity-me mode. Now I was moving. Now I had belief. Now I had relief. Now I had hope.

No question I thought it would kill me at times, but I kept coming back. Even when a change in Ellen's work schedule forced her to shift her workout time, leaving me alone in that class, I stayed with it. I did what I could do, and when I couldn't, I stopped and went over and sat on the bike for a while. That became my spot, back in the corner, by the bike. Everyone who's ever done aerobics knows what I mean by my "spot." It's your place in the room, the same place you do your thing every day. You own it. Everyone knows and respects each other's spot in an aerobics room, and nobody messes with someone else's spot.

My spot was back in the corner, by the bike, the fan,

and the water fountain. Day after day that's where I went, ignoring the smirks, sideways glances, and looks of pity from some of my classmates. One day, the owner of the club, Gigi herself, passed me in the hall and greeted me by name. "Hi, Dee," she said. That's it. Two little words. But to me, it was as if the heavens had opened. No way can words do justice to what that did for my self-esteem. Here was Gigi herself, tall, thin as a rail, zero percent body fat, a resting heart rate of forty-two — I mean, the woman was just *it*. Fit, fit, *fit*. And she knew who I was. She knew my name. And she took the trouble to stop and say hi.

Let me tell you, I took that little dinky "Hi" and I made it into a mountain. My security mountain. My self-esteem mountain. I turned that tiny little crumb into something I could cling to, something to build on until another crumb came my way.

And they kept coming, those crumbs. Some of my classmates began treating me as though I belonged, once I showed them I was there to stay. Instructors began paying attention, giving me adjusted patterns and movements to fit the restrictions of my body. At home, my eating habits were no longer compulsive.

I noticed there were no more episodes of getting up at midnight and raiding the refrigerator. I ate the cookies, but I didn't lie about who ate them. I didn't feel the need to lie because I wasn't eating the whole package anymore. I was eating reasonable amounts.

My mood and energy were much improved, too. I wasn't spending most of the day on the couch watching the tube. I would venture outside and swing and play with the boys. I kept the house up on a regular basis, and I found I wasn't biting Keith's head off for being late (which happens more often than not). Keith even noticed the happier, cheerier Dee.

I was still obese, but that wasn't my focus anymore. I was thinking about my next workout, anticipating the fun, yet still a bit apprehensive. It was such a delight to have something else to think about, to work on, other than *eating*. This "trying" thing was really steering my preoccupation with food and misery into something else. Something was in motion here, and it felt good. No longer did I feel the urge to step on a scale, as I had done compulsively whenever I was on a diet.

The scale. Thank God I was finally out of that trap. Think about it. The scale can be such a monster. You don't want to come near one when you're fat — I mean, you might as well just go get a gun and shoot yourself as step on a scale to see how overweight you are, especially when you weigh as much as I did — over three hundred pounds.

The bottom line on the whole scales-and-weight thing was, after about 280 pounds, I just didn't care or pay attention to the numbers. I lost about seventeen pounds after my second son was born, but I gained that back right away and more. When the 5X shirt I had and the one black elastic skirt I owned started not to fit, the only thing I had left that would fit over my body was a single pink coverup. What kind of masochist would want to keep track at that point?

I did check in on the weight thing whenever I saw my doctor — I *had* to — and that process in itself was humiliating. I was too large for his scales to measure — no scale's needle even goes that far — so we had to estimate my weight. His guess was that I was anywhere from 310 to 340, at my largest.

Let me tell you, I wasn't exactly in a picture-taking mood. I was so ashamed and felt so bad and was so *big* I could barely move. I'd had it with scales, and for good reason. I'd been a slave to the scale long enough. You're a slave to the scale when you're on a diet, measuring your life by those little one-pound lines, and where does it get you? How traditional is that? And, in most cases, how fruitless is it?

No, for the first time in my life I was going to do something about my body without letting that little piece of tin dictate my direction.

I was excited, and being me, Ms. Enthusiasm, I carried that excitement into my OA meetings, gushing about the wonders exercise was doing with my life. I realized that by moving my body I was moving my mind. And the strokes, those crumbs of confidence, were actually empowering me to pat myself on the back, to become my own best cheering section. It was becoming more clear to me how much mind and body really do work together. I was becoming my own best friend, too!

My new approach to this process of rearranging my reason for getting this activity habit and keeping it was lightening up the entire rest of my life. It was activity heaven. It was empowering-my-body-and-brain heaven. It was setting me *free*!

Imagine my shock when my glee was met by my OA group with silence and raised eyebrows.

I was basically told that it was wrong to bring outside stuff into those meetings. If it wasn't part of the twelve steps, part of the program, it didn't belong. That really surprised me, the exclusivity. I was really disappointed, because OA had done so much for me. I had gotten so much out of it, so many valuable tools. But when they warned me not to talk too much about exercise, I thought about the fact that all we *did* talk about was food — about our obsession and preoccupation with food. And it dawned on me that even there, even in the OA setting, we were still trapped, still limited, by the focus on eating. I really wanted to look beyond that. I needed to look beyond it.

When I had begun attending the OA meetings, I had no tools whatsoever with which to work effectively on my problems with food and weight. Thanks to OA, I was able to start to develop some of those tools — self-perspective, self-esteem, self-confidence — strengths that, ironically, allowed me the courage to finally leave the group a year after I joined it, to begin my new journey into health and fitness.

I have so much to thank OA for. I learned an enormous amount about myself and about my eating habits. Most of all, I came to understand that I had used food all my life the way other people use drugs or alcohol. Or sex. Or their job. Or anything in their life that becomes an addiction because they're turning to it as an escape from something they don't want to or are unable to face.

Those addictions all come from basically the same place, that pressure place, that need-to-feel-accepted place, that trying-to-be-the-best place, and the only way out is to find a tool that works. For me, those tools became writing — which I'd done on and off during the good times, all my life; the friends I'd made in this new home I'd found, the fitness center; and most of all, the pursuit of fitness itself: *exercise*.

That "way out" comes not just from finding a tool but from finding and using a new, better, less destructive tool with which to cope. Let's face it. As I stated before, we all cope. We all use different tools to do it. It's when our coping tools take over and monopolize and control us rather than help us that the imbalance occurs. They're no longer tools if they're in charge.

By the end of 1990, after a year at Gigi's, I was a little disappointed, a little taken aback that my body size hadn't seemed to change. I'd actually lost thirty pounds, a sizable amount on the face of it, but that was only a mere sliver of the three-hundred-plus I'd begun at.

I had mixed feelings about my journey thus far. With a lifetime of "getting there quick" being the mental mind-set for success, there was very little out there rewarding me for the "process," for the idea that progress was success, that those first thirty pounds could be my first gold medal. That's what I tried to keep telling myself, yet everywhere I looked, that was *not* being reinforced or recognized. What I saw almost everywhere I turned was the claim that the "quick fix" was the only success, that there was no glory in the process.

Let me tell you about one incident that illustrates this so well. One of the directors in the program I eventually developed told me how her mother had begun attending water exercise classes in another city. She was too intimidated to take them in her own town, where her daughter was a great fitness instructor. When she told her daughter about her first two weeks of classes, the daughter's reply was, "Well, Mom, you start and stop this stuff all the time. You have to go longer than two weeks to get anywhere."

I stopped her right there and said, "You mean you didn't send your mom a dozen roses? She comes to you to tell you about her attempt, to get some positive strokes, some affirmation, and you jam her like that?"

Wow, did the lights come on in this person's eyes. She broke down in tears right there on the spot, realizing that all this time her mother was reaching out to her for approval, for those crumbs of positive reinforcement, which she could then turn into confidence and staying power, and what did she get from her daughter? The usual "Oh, this again. So you've started. So you're trying. So what? That's not good enough."

Let me tell you, and I'll say it a thousand times if I say it once, "IT'S GOOD ENOUGH!" Trying is the key to everything. It's the key to life. It's the key to health. It's the key to happiness.

That first thirty pounds I lost at Gigi's might not have seemed like much, but the fact was, when I took the time to examine it, that I could now do things that I hadn't done in years. I could play with my boys and not even break a sweat. I could go sixteen hours a day, get out of the house, visit friends, shop, work out, *live*. So what if I was still overweight, I thought, this was definitely different.

Something was really changing, and it had nothing to do with fixating on food. My eating habits were changing, but it was happening gradually, *naturally*. My behaviors were shifting, like noticing that I was full and not feeling the need to keep stuffing my face. I noticed that I did not have to clean my plate when I was full. I really started to pay attention to how I felt, and I actually started to enjoy the taste of the food and not just feel the need to cram it in so I wouldn't miss out on that last drop or bite, as if the world would end if I didn't get all that food on that plate into my mouth. This is where I began looking at my behaviors and habits about food and became aware of them.

I allowed myself to eat whatever and whenever I felt like it, but I no longer felt like it as often as I used to. I no longer *needed* to eat the way I had before. I was aware of what was happening, aware of what I was and wasn't eating, but I didn't get hyper-diligent. I didn't get carried away and start pushing it. The place I did my pushing was in that aerobics room, and I let the rest take care of itself. I had a long journey ahead of me, and I could sense that this was the way to begin.

That aerobics room. It was life-saving for me just to show up. The music, the energy, Ellen — this was my oasis, my pleasure palace, a bright spot no matter how light or dark the rest of my day might be.

I'm just talking about the place, never mind what I could or couldn't *do* in it. And in the beginning I couldn't do much. I started out being able to do maybe three or four minutes at a time of marching in place, if I was lucky. Then I'd have to stop, take a break. Marching in place, Step-Touching, Grapevines — basic aerobic moves, or *my* version of basic aerobic moves — in the beginning I'd make up rough imitations of what the others were doing. The pros call it "modifications," but I didn't know that term. I called it "faking it." And sometimes I'd fall off the pace, or get lost, or run out of gas, and I'd just stop, wait a while, and jump back in when I was ready. Sure I felt frustrated.

Sure I got a little upset sometimes. Sure I felt self-conscious and intimidated. But I kept *trying*. I was committed like never before in my life, and that made all the difference in the world.

As I got to learn the moves more and my body began developing a bit, the process really started kicking in. Anybody of any size, shape, color, or gender can do what I did. Anyone can be a part of this. The moves? Simple. Can you take your right foot to the right and have your left foot join it, then take your left foot to the left and have your right foot join it? That's called a Step-Touch. Simple.

Don't be put off or intimidated by all the terminology and jargon. It's like anything else, it's just words. Get past the language and it's no big deal. Don't let those words be some big, forbidding wall.

And don't worry about the pace or power of the people doing *their* versions of the Step-Touch around you. Who cares if you're doing it slower or a little differently than everyone else? You're *doing* it, and that will yield results. That will make a difference in your life. The thousand-and-one little adjustments you might need to make to fit the movements and exercises to the specifics of your body and your abilities and your sensitivities and limitations and uniqueness are not liabilities. They are not something to be self-conscious about. Quite the contrary, they are something to take pride and pleasure in. They are the keys that can unlock the door into a room you might have assumed you could never enter — the room of fitness.

By the end of that first year I'd seen incredible changes in my body's ability to simply move. I was more flexible, I had more endurance, I was doing the moves those around

me were doing, and at the same pace they were doing them
at. Whereas in the beginning I could hardly lift my feet to
slide them side to side, now I was crossing my steps, literally bouncing with energy . . . dancing! Who would have
dreamed it?

If I had any doubts about how far I'd come in one short
year, they were erased that December when, caught up in
the Christmas rush, I stopped working out for three weeks.
What happened? The old programming kicked in. I re-
gressed, started stuffing myself again, got bitchy, began
complaining. Finally Keith told me one day to take a long
hike off a short pier.

"You're a nightmare," he said. And he was right. I was
even worse than I'd been before, and that was when I knew
how much I needed what I was getting out of that workout
room, not for my body or my appearance or how other
people felt about me, but for how I felt about *myself,* for
how happy it made me and how happy that made the people around me, the people I loved.

I returned to Gigi's that January with a vengeance. I
thought every day about how my life was changing, and
that led to thinking about how other lives, lives like my
own, could be changed in the same way.

I thought to myself, How many other people would
come to a place like this, a hardbody studio, if they knew
they'd be accepted and embraced regardless of whether
they could dance and jump around the room at the rate of
the workout animals around them?

I thought about the past year and everything I'd been
through and how I would have loved to have even one or
two people give me the time of day during those first

couple of months, how I would have loved one of the instructors to reach out to me sooner and meet me at my limits and work with me from there, give me something to go on so I could start getting somewhere rather than just sitting it out if I couldn't keep up, or faking it, or figuring it out on my own and doing the best I could.

I would have loved having an instructor like that. And then I thought, Why not *me*? Why can't I do what they're doing, with a class full of people like myself?

That's what I came in to ask Gigi the next day:

"Why can't *I* be an instructor?"

7

If I Could Do That...

When I showed up at the studio that January with the notion of becoming an instructor, the reaction of Gigi and her staff was predictable. Part supportive, mostly disbelieving. Neat idea, Dee. Pat the little doggie on the head. You're so adorable. I got a lot of that. On the other hand, I also heard, Gee, that's a *great* idea. You might really be on to something. There was definitely some support there, especially on Gigi's part, but I could feel — and even hear — the undercurrents among some of the staff that the idea of my becoming an instructor was so unthinkable to them it was beyond ridiculous. They didn't take it seriously enough to say it was ridiculous. It was more that they thought it was *cute.*

No matter. I wasn't looking for a vote on this thing. With some steering from Gigi, I enrolled in a National Dance and Exercise Instructor Training Association

(NDEITA) workshop, part of which included a written exam required of all entry-level aerobic instructors. The day of the test, I arrived at the Lake Charles YMCA, where I was one of about thirty men and women ushered into an empty tile-floored classroom.

My fellow test-takers were mostly athletic-looking people, very much in shape. There were a couple of older women with little pot bellies, probably there so they could be certified to teach water aerobics, something low-low-level. But there was no one anywhere *near* my size. Of course I got a few looks, as always. Good for you, honey. Sure it bothered me, but I tried to treat it as nothing more than water off my back. I was there for one thing, to ace that test.

Which I did. The day-long exam, including some rudimentary physical workouts along with the written test, which covered basic physiology and kinesiology as well as introductory training techniques, was a snap. The next morning I was at Gigi's office door with a perfect score in hand.

"All right, Gigi," I said. "Let's go."

She couldn't believe it. Her encouragement up to that point had come more from affection than from truly believing I was going to get anywhere with this scheme. Now she was faced with something she hadn't imagined she'd have to deal with, and so she tossed it back in my court, turning it into put-your-money-where-your-mouth-is time by telling me if I could get ten people to sign up for a month, she'd give it a try. If I found the bodies, she said, she'd give me a room and a time slot to try teaching them.

So I made up my own flyers, got them printed, and

went around to every Weight Watchers location, every plus-size clothing shop, every grocery store in town, taping up these announcements, introducing a brand-new, low-low-*very*-low-intensity pre-aerobics workout specifically for overweight people, *taught* by an overweight instructor.

Then I sat back and prayed for a response.

I got it. A month after the flyers went up, twelve prospects had signed up, all of them women. And so, on a Monday morning in April 1991, I walked into a workout studio at Gigi's and for the first time stepped to the front of the class rather than to the rear.

I could see Gigi and some of the others hanging around out in the lobby, looking in through the door, getting a load of the misfits, the little fat class. I said a silent little prayer to myself, popped my "Got to Git" music tape into the machine, punched the play button . . . and . . . kicked . . . aerobic . . . butt.

I'm telling you, it was like magic, moving from helping myself to actually sharing with others what was doing so much for me. It felt so good to be in front of that class, motivating them, making them smile, helping them feel accepted, feel comfortable, feel that they belonged, because they *did!* Watching their faces light up and seeing them smile and laugh as they moved their bodies. I realized at that moment I didn't have to wear a thong to belong, and neither did my class. We could move our bodies and do our own thing and have fun and feel good. No, feel great, feel INCREDIBLE! The smiles, the laughter, the ease, the pure, unadulterated, mega-encouraging *joy* kept expanding as the music played and our bodies moved.

It was one of the most memorable hours of my life,

that first class. It was an hour that went by like a minute. I'm telling you, it was amazing.

And it wouldn't have worked if my students hadn't seen a woman their own size busting her moves in front of those mirrors. They told me so. If I could do that, they said, then by God, so could they. I heard that so many times, over and over again. I still hear it.

Beyond the sheer inspiration and identification, what set my class apart was the specialized attention I gave each student from the second they came through that door, assessing their abilities and adjusting various techniques to meet their limitations. No one in that room was going to have to bail out, sit on a bike, and just watch.

That's the thing about a true aerobics workout. There's no need to bust a gut, no need to "feel the burn," no need to pump and pant like a crazed animal. I mean, that kind of madly choreographed 78 r.p.m. *Flashdance* stuff is fine if you're up to it. But you don't have to do that to give your body what it needs. And I don't have to do that to guide you through a workout that will give you, your heart, and your muscles everything they need in terms of exercise. All I've got to do is keep you moving in a zone that will effect aerobic capacity, that will have your heart pumping in a healthy, effective way. That's all I've got to do.

According to the ACSM (American College of Sports Medicine) guidelines for cardiovascular training, the typical person in exercise should work within 60 to 90 percent of his or her maximum heart rate. For myself and the students I begin with, I prefer working at a range between 60 and 70 percent. What I have my students do is measure their heart rate by taking their pulse in either their wrist or their neck (your wrist is where your radial artery is located; your carotid artery is in your neck). Using your first two fingers — not your thumb, because your thumb may actually have a small pulse in it — press to the point where you can feel a pulse, start at zero, and count the number of pulses you feel in 10 seconds. The goal is about 24 pulses in that period, which equals roughly 144 pulses a minute, which is roughly a 70 percent range of intensity — just what we're after. That's all we need to achieve. We don't have to go to 90 percent. We don't have to kill the cow to change our lives and help ourselves.

If you're in the aerobics studio, doing your workout, and you want to throw in fancy arm movements, great. If you can start jumping, actually getting off the ground after a while, super. But you don't need to do any of that to change your body, to start affecting the flow of your blood and the strength of your breath. All you've got to do is move, and all I've got to do is *keep* you moving.

With the classes I had, the ones I still have — people who have been discouraged and frustrated by fitness, who have come to see it as something completely out of their reach, who are full of doubt and skepticism when they edge into an aerobics room — I've got to make it *fun* and I've got to make it work. I've got to have them taste success that very first day, the very first time they walk through those doors, because if it doesn't work, if they feel like a failure, there won't be a second time. I'll never see them again. When they walk through the door that first day, all the chips are on the table. I've only got one chance, that's it.

There were already low-impact classes at Gigi's, instructors guiding routines designed for the same over-weight, older, and underconditioned students I was aiming at. But membership in those classes was sparse. The approach to the students was not specialized, not individually tailored. And, most of all, the instructors were not over-weight or older — they were the same lean, mean aerobic machines leading the hardbody classes next door.

Why did my class catch fire when those others didn't? There were a lot of reasons, but I'd say it basically boiled down to sensitivity and understanding, to breaking down the barrier between the instructor and the student, break-ing down the gap that can seem so huge between a person who's totally out of condition and the perfectly condi-tioned, streamlined "fit" person in front of that room.

It's all a matter of motivation, of believing, of breaking through and connecting, of getting that tantalizing taste of success, no matter how small it is, and building on that. And having fun in the process.

Motivation. What exactly is that? For me, motivation means action. If I am motivated, I act. I do. I move, whether it's physically or mentally. And when you act or do or move, guess what? Change happens. That is a fact. Mo-tivation in its truest form is action. If I am truly motivated, I will act. I will *do*. Where "believing" comes in is taking motivation on and on and on to create "staying power."

Think about this. Have you ever made New Year's reso-lutions? Of course you have. We all have, at one time or an-other. Now ask yourself, have you ever made the same resolution over and over again? Now why did you do that? Why have *I* done that? Every year I made that New Year's resolution to start that diet, to start that exercise, and you know what? I spent many a year making the same dang resolution over again. I would start out motivated, stay with it a couple of weeks, then lose it. I started thinking about why I didn't keep the resolution going, why I didn't keep that motivation going, and you know what I came up with? I didn't keep the resolution because I didn't believe I *deserved* it! If I had taken my motivation one step further and worked on *believing I deserved this,* I would have stuck with it.

I've got absolutely no doubt about it. Believing is the key to staying power, and believing is directly linked to how I feel about myself and my body, what the experts call "body image." And the key thing to understand about body image — *healthy* body image — is that it has nothing to do with anyone else's image of your body, which of course is one of the major lures that lead us all down the dead-end paths of eating disorders. A healthy body image begins and ends with your image of your own body, and that image has nothing to do with your body's physical size, shape, or appearance. It has everything to do with how you feel about your body, which has everything to do with how you feel about yourself.

Can you imagine anything more liberating than this, to be freed from the trap of judging yourself, condemning yourself, punishing and pushing yourself based on standards set by some imaginary "other"? To make that shift, from looking through the eyes of others to seeing and caressing yourself through your own eyes, is like stepping into an entirely new existence. Veils are lifted. Shadows slide away. Enormous pressures and weights disappear, replaced by a sense of sunshine and freedom and possibility. There was a book (and a movie) that came out a few years back called *The Unbearable Lightness of Being.* That's a great phrase to describe the feeling that comes with breaking the shackles of an unhealthy body image, with taking charge of your own sense of your self.

I deserve it. That phrase can't be repeated enough. It's the source of true motivation, the center of staying power, the key to success.

I deserve it. Say it. Believe it. And you'll be on your way to fitness in the fullest sense of the word.

We said it, and believed it, over and over again in my classes at Gigi's, and word began spreading, not just to the new students who began filling my roster, but to some of the other instructors, several of whom came in and sampled my class, lining up alongside my students, to see just what it was that was working so well for me. They wanted to check this situation out.

I'll never forget my friend Cathy Seal coming in one morning — a beautiful sandy blonde with a killer body, one of Gigi's instructors. Cathy came in, took my class, and walked up to me at the end totally amazed. "Dee," she told me, "you just gave me a great workout!"

I can't tell you what that did, not just for me, but for my students. The pride, the self-esteem in that entire room, just went through the ceiling.

We knew we were real. We were sweating just like real people sweat. We were fit, each in his or her own way. Our sweat in that room was no different from the sweat of the thong-clad hardbodies at the 5:30 class, and, in fact, those hardbodies could share their sweat in the same workout room with us. Thus began the breakdown of those walls and barriers and misconceptions about what and who can own fitness, of who is allowed to be fit and who is not. We weren't just the "exercise class for misfits" anymore. We were an exercise class for people just like every other class at that club.

That was such an important key to my program, that my students felt included, that they felt they belonged, that they were a part of this fitness center just like everyone else. There are plenty of programs aimed at the under-conditioned across America, both inside centers like Gigi's and at nursing homes, hospitals, and fat farms all over the country — programs geared toward the ill, the overweight, and the elderly. But those programs are set apart, isolated, ghettoized, and many of the students in them feel that way. That ghettoization, I firmly believe, is yet another reason that so many people simply stay away.

Belonging. That is *so* important. Like a coyote belonging to the pack, like a newborn baby belonging to his or her family, a sense of security, a sense of fulfillment or having purpose, being of substance — all of these things stem from that basic comfort of belonging. It's about love and acceptance of *you,* unconditionally, based on no requirements other than the fact that you are who you are and that is what matters most. To belong is to have meaning. It is the essence of the soul. It feeds the soul and the heart and the body and the mind. Belonging validates acceptance. As humans, whether we admit it consciously or not, whether we are cognizant of it or not, we all need to belong. Belonging fills us and brings peace and serenity. It can armor us with courage and strength to face the complexities and challenges of life.

Belonging, in one way or another, in one space or another, in one place or another, is an essential part of being alive. Feeling like you're somewhere on that spectrum with everybody else, even if you're way out at the end of it. Being connected to the "normal" world, being in the same setting, doing the same thing, feeling like you're part of the same world as everyone else.

That's what I made a point of showing and sharing at Gigi's: that we might look different and have different limitations than the aerobic animals, that we might be doing our thing at a different rate and in a different way than they were, but we were on the exact same path they were on, aiming at the same goal and committed to nothing less than achieving it — that goal, of course, being fitness. True, total, complete, inside-and-out, life-improving, life-affirming, aim-at-the-contents-and-let-the-container-take-care-of-itself *fitness.*

By the beginning of 1992, less than a year after I began offering them, enrollment in my classes had swelled to more than two hundred — bumping total membership at Gigi's club by more than a fourth. I was spending almost every day of the week at the club, teaching morning and evening classes, meeting the demands of students who seemed to be crawling out of the woodwork.

As those demands grew, so did my knowledge of my students' needs — needs that began extending beyond the bounds of the workout room. It was when I began responding to those needs that my program leaped to a completely new level in terms of both breadth and depth.

It was also at that point that I began meeting resistance from the last place in the world I would have expected it — my own husband, Keith.

This Train Is Leaving

It was after my evening sessions, my last class of each night, that I began a little ritual with a handful of my students. A half dozen of them, maybe more, would sit around with me, lingering, towels draped around our necks, our shirts soaked with sweat, no one in a rush to get home, all of us simply hanging out in a hallway, in a locker room, wherever, the conversation fast and free-flowing, focused on the stuff of our lives, the day-to-day context that framed the time we were spending at Gigi's.

We'd talk about the bad week that we'd had, or we'd talk about something good that had happened. These weren't all "fat" things we were gabbing about, but that was the predominant theme — the hundreds of day-to-day challenges and struggles only an overweight person can understand.

Every night we'd wind up hanging out like that, a few

more people joining us every week, all of us talking until they shut out the lights and locked the doors. The great thing was, these weren't just bitch sessions, a bunch of unhappy, overweight women sitting around complaining about how crappy their lives were and how unfair the world was. Everything about these conversations was positive and constructive. It was invigorating, just like the workout we'd just finished.

It didn't take me long to see that these post-workout get-togethers could — should — become a part of the program, a formalized support session of sorts. I didn't want it to be a Weight Watchers thing. I didn't want it to be an OA thing. But I wanted to take it a step beyond just sitting around and rapping. A lot of questions came up in those discussions — questions about nutrition, diets, trends in health and fitness, theories about body image, an article somebody had read in the newspaper or a magazine, a program someone had seen on TV — and I realized how worthwhile it would be, beyond the basic sense of connection and bonding and belonging that was clearly so rewarding about those "hangout" sessions, to start bringing back some answers.

I had been continuing to push my own boundaries, in terms of both education and credentials. I had started studying and training for the American Council on Exercise (ACE) aerobic instructor's examination, a far more demanding and prestigious test than the entry-level NDEITA exam I had passed a year earlier. ACE certification was the doorway into the arena of full-time professional aerobics instruction. Even as I studied for that test, I began taking steps toward extending my class beyond the workout room.

I asked Gigi if there was a room we could have for an extra hour every night. Hanging out in the hall wasn't going to make it anymore, not for what I had in mind. She said she didn't have anything, so I said what about the dressing room? I would rather have had something a little nicer, but I took what we could get. And so that's where the "classes" started — in the dressing room.

We gathered every week, I and a dozen or so of my students. I or one of them would bring in the title of a book we all might want to read, or an article I'd Xerox and pass around to everyone there. We'd share that information, take it home, read it, and gather the following week to discuss it. Nobody was God. Nobody was the leader. Yes, they turned to me a lot, and I took on the responsibility of becoming as much of an authority as I could, but this wasn't about anyone being a control freak. We were all in this together, all of us with things we didn't know, all of us with things to learn.

I became a handout junkie. Gigi had a wall of handouts; I got the idea from her. Pretty soon I had a virtual library going, with Xeroxes of articles on everything from low-intensity weight training to plus-size clothing, from the latest studies on diabetes or arthritis to trends in homeopathic medicine. And I also began to invite experts to come in and speak to the group.

I'm not a dietitian. I wasn't going to play dietitian. But could I link up with a registered dietitian who would come in and help us? Why not? The same with doctors and counselors who specialized in eating disorders. Or physiologists. Or physical therapists. Or chiropractors. Or meditation instructors. Or body image experts, people in the clothing business, or the cosmetics business, even hairdressers. Anyone with something to offer in the way of expertise and advice for some of the specific needs and desires of the members of our group, that's whom I reached out to.

And they came. Of course they came. I mean, figure it out. If anybody in our group wound up needing something any of these experts had to offer, what were they more apt to do — go hunting through the flipping yellow pages or call one of these people whose names they already knew and who had already made themselves available, who had already donated the time to come and share what they knew with us.

For many of the women in my classes, these meetings, this entire program, became the bedrock of their lives, something around which they planned their entire week. And their connection to one another didn't stop at the gym. We created a phone list, so if someone was in a crisis, or whatever, if they just wanted to reach out to a friend and talk, then they could pick up the phone and dial. They weren't isolated.

It was almost too good to be true, the momentum we started picking up, the attention we began receiving from the local media there in Lake Charles, from the newspaper and the television stations. There was a hint of jealousy from Gigi, but I expected that. What I did not expect was the resistance I began to face from the last person I thought would be unhappy about what I was doing — my husband, Keith.

When I first started all this, he was happy I was doing

it, happy I was picking myself up from the pits I'd been in for so long. But then, when things really began rolling, when it was clear how committed I was to this, that something was really changing here, I started hearing little comments from him, like, "Oh, you're going to the Fat Club again?"

That blew me over. I mean, how ironic is that: here this man would marry me and I'd been big all my life, unhealthy and almost always unhappy, and now I was trying to do something about it, breaking through, getting healthier, feeling happier. I'm going to live longer, I'm going to be a better mom for my kids, a better wife for him — all those things are starting to happen and what do I get from him? Smartass remarks. Sarcasm.

It would have made more sense if he'd called me names and made fun of me back when I was fat and doing nothing about it. Now I was trying to change my life for the better, and *now* he was giving me a hard time.

Keith's complaints only got worse as my program expanded into its "educational" sphere, moving out of the workout room and into those end-of-the-night group sessions. Now it was "Oh, you've got that damn thing tonight. So you'll be down there at nine-thirty this morning and I won't see you until eleven-thirty tonight?"

I understood by then what was going on, that this wasn't just happening with me. I was hearing it from more than a few of my students, that the very people they thought would be excited and ecstatic and the most supportive of their making themselves healthier wound up often being the most resistant.

It's about change. It's about what change does to a relationship — any relationship that's been going on for a
long time. The way people stay together in this life is by figuring out how to fit with each other, how to find a balance,
an equilibrium in their lives that allows them to accept and
coexist with the other person. Each partner makes space
for and adjusts to the other's habits, nuances, quirks,
strengths, weaknesses. There are a million ways people
find that balance, but in one way or another, the ones who
have been together for a good amount of time do find it.

Which brings up the challenge of change. Because if
people make a change in themselves, a shift of any sort,
then chances are that's going to upset the balance. There's
going to have to be an adjustment on the part of the other
person as well, so they can stay in balance, and that's not
always easy, and it's often pretty scary.

The change might be about getting a life, getting a career . . . or it might be about one partner finally getting up
off the couch and taking her health into her hands. Whatever it is, if the other person isn't ready to make some
changes, too, then as often as not you're going to have
some problems. You're going to see one person digging in
their heels and holding on to what they know. They're going to cling to the way things have always been, and they're
going to try to get you to cling to it, too.

That's what happened with Keith. All he'd ever known
was me being fat, me being unhealthy and generally unhappy, me being home on the sofa, with him whenever he
was there. There was a certain comfort and security in
that. But now I wasn't there all the time. Now I had some-

thing else I cared about, some place else I was spending some of my time. I was still home when I was supposed to be, still taking care of all my responsibilities as a mother to my boys and a wife to Keith. As a matter of fact, I was doing those things better than ever, because I now had more energy and motivation to do them. But there was something else that was important to me now as well, and Keith was afraid of that. It was threatening to him. He felt as though he was being pushed aside and maybe he wouldn't matter to me anymore. Way out there was the idea that I might actually get thin and leave him. He felt that, too, even though he never came right out and said it.

It was about that time that one of my favorite students, a woman named Mona, shared with me what she was going through with her husband, something much like what I was getting from Keith.

Every one of my students is special, truly beautiful. I really feel that way. But Mona was beyond special. She was about five years older than I was, with four children, very well off. She and her husband owned their own welding business. They had a nice house, boats, all of that.

Mona was big. *Big* big. Bigger than I was. She weighed three thirty, maybe three fifty when we first met. A beautiful woman, with brown hair, green eyes, perfect complexion, a gorgeous face, and she dressed very, very well, all the best from the plus-size shops. She could afford it.

Mona had always had a weight problem. Her parents had a history of diabetes and heart disease, too, so she entered the program with a lot of needs. And it clicked right from the beginning. I mean, her personality was so perfect, so enthusiastic, so into it. She was rocking and rolling right from the start.

I get as personal as I can with all my students, while still remaining professional. Everyone has my phone number, and they know they can call me anytime. But with Mona, our personal relationship went even further. I kind of took her under my wing, went to her house, our husbands met, our kids played.

So it hit me all the harder when Mona suddenly started missing a class here and there, then a couple in a row, then she started hardly coming at all. I asked her what was going on, was anything wrong, and at first she wouldn't say. But finally she told me it was her husband. He had started getting on her.

"You're not cooking dinner."

"You're going out four nights a week exercising now instead of three."

"You've got the kids to take care of."

These were the things Mona's husband was saying to her. It got to the point where he became ugly, really mean, and she couldn't take the pressure. They were fighting all the time. It was disrupting the family, the kids. Finally she had to make a choice between her marriage and my classes, and that was it. No more Mona.

It was several months before I heard from her again. Her weight had gone back up, way up. She was almost bedridden because of diabetes.

It broke my heart, what happened to Mona, because I know I could have helped her.

Mona is not alone. So many women wind up in her situation and are forced by their spouses to make a choice. I faced that choice myself, but there was no question in my mind what the decision was going to be, not a flicker of in-decision or doubt. I told Keith, "Hey, I'm doing this, like it or lump it. You can either get along with me or you can not get along with me, but I am *doing* this.

"You're on this train or not," I told him, "but either way, it is leaving the station."

9

Lady Liberty

Keith stayed on that train, and it pulled out. Enrollment in my classes really started to snowball, and I kept pace, adding to my own knowledge and credentials to keep ahead of the growing demands of my students. The ACE exam, along with certification as a personal trainer, not only gave me top-level credentials, but provided me with a wealth of hands-on knowledge I could bring back and apply to my special students.

These exams were extremely comprehensive — kinesiology, biomechanics, nutrition, CPR, bone structure, muscle synergistic groups, heart rate monitoring, stroke volume, anaerobic versus aerobic conditioning — you've really got to know your stuff. I'm not saying you need to be a rocket scientist, but if you don't study this stuff and study hard, you're not going to make it. I know as many people who have taken these tests and failed as have taken them and passed. This is heavy-duty material, no doubt about it.

I had always been a good student, thank God, and now it was no different. I passed those tests with strong scores, and that sent me back into the workout studio with even more energy and confidence than ever. We were *all* rockin' and rollin' in the self-esteem department. Think about it. I didn't have the background of these other instructors. I hadn't been an athlete in school, or a cheerleader, or a dancer. I'd never been a ballerina. I was fat most of my life, just trying to survive, and now, all of a sudden, I'm breaking into the fitness world and bing-bang-boom, here I am, a fitness professional. What's a tendon? What's a ligament? Oh, muscle innervation? Let me tell you about muscle innervation.

For me, even more than for my fellow instructors, this knowledge was crucially connected to the program I was still continuing to shape in the workout room, responding to the specific physical needs and limitations of my students. If you don't understand the human body, how it functions both as a piece of machinery and as a living thing, then you have no basis or frame of reference to create safe and effective exercise, especially for the kinds of students I had.

For example, when you're dealing with somebody with rheumatoid arthritis, you've got to understand and be aware of the fact that pain is a part of their life, a constant reality every minute of the day, and you have to understand where that pain comes from, why they feel it, how pain is going to be a part of the physical activity you'll be asking them to do in that workout room, and how much pain is safe.

I had each new student fill out a detailed health history form, so I could identify and really zero in on their individual conditions, limitations, and needs. I remember one woman in particular who came in with a history of arthritis. I said to her, "Debbie, by the way, I want you to know I'm aware of the fact that you will experience some pain in here, and what I'd like you to do is to give me an idea of what's normal for you."

Do you have any idea how she heard those simple words? This woman wanted to marry me, she was so elated. She'd tried aerobics before, and no one had ever asked about her pain. It had always been her problem to deal with. This was the first time she'd stepped into a situation like this and had somebody actually acknowledge what she was facing, what she was going through. It was as if somebody was relating to her for the first time, as if somebody knew her.

As my program grew, both I and my students felt the growing need to measure the results of our efforts. It's only natural. Yes, we felt better physically, emotionally, even spiritually in terms of our connections to one another. But we were nagged by that basic need to quantify our progress, to see in a tangible way how we were doing, how our bodies were changing.

I thought back to everything I'd learned, both through personal experience and through hearing so many others' stories, and I knew the one thing *not* to measure was pounds. How long had I been a slave to the scale, and how many times did it break my heart and my spirit? I thought about how it shocked me my first year at Gigi's, how it really set me back when I stepped on the scale and saw how little weight I'd lost. I had pulled out the tape measure and could see I'd lost three inches in the waist, but I still weighed nearly as much as I had at the start. And why was that? Did I know then that part of the conditioning process is that muscle begins to replace fat, and muscle is denser than fat, that it weighs more than fat, and so you can actually lose fat and yet not be losing weight, at least not initially?

No, I did not know that then. But I knew it now. And I thought to myself, let's look at how our clothes are hanging looser on ourselves, how we're fitting into smaller sizes. Forget the scale. Let's take out the tape measure. If we want to look at numbers, let's look at inches, not pounds.

And that's when I got the idea of the parties. A group celebration. Every ninety days. Each person's measurements would be charted over the course of those three months, then we would all come together in a festive setting where each person, every single one, would be recognized for their progress, no matter how small or large it had been.

Like so much else I was doing, this was about breaking those old patterns. In this case, it was that cycle of disappointment and defeat, the jumping on the scale and saying, Wow, I bet I've lost ten pounds, and it turns out you've lost maybe three. If that happens, do you praise the Lord and give yourself a pat on the back and treat yourself to a hot bubble bath for the good work you've done? Do you even know what you've done? Oh no, you go crucify yourself and slink back to the kitchen and eat a gallon of ice cream and sabotage a month and a half of good stuff because you didn't lose the number of pounds you thought you should have.

It was that old syndrome of the glass half empty versus the glass half full. I needed to somehow keep my students focused on what they had achieved, not what they hadn't. I was pounding them with information, continuing to broaden the educational and awareness aspects of my program, making sure we all understood and realized what was happening inside our bodies as well as outside. With that, with all we were doing both in the workout room and outside it, I launched yet another prong of my program — the "Celebrations."

This was just another extension, another tool, another way of making this pursuit of fitness part of our entire environment. The more we take fitness out of the workout room and integrate it into our daily lives, the more we're going to make that magic. This becomes an integral part of our lives, not just something we do an hour a day, three or four days a week, not just something we do at the gym, not just something that's for ourselves, but something that includes these people who are now sharing this experience with us, these people who are now our friends.

Each Celebration was a party. One every ninety days. Everyone comes. Everyone gets recognized. We included the families at these parties, too. Absolutely. Because this is about inclusion, not exclusion. It's about everyone who's a part of your life being a part of what's happening with and to you, because they are a part of it, whether they realize it or not. This sense of inclusion, by the way, in many cases, speaks directly to that problem of resistance so many people who get into fitness face from their spouses or significant others.

Everybody's a part of this. One gathering might be a canoeing outing. Or rafting. Bowling maybe. Or a formal banquet. Pony rides for the kids. Photographs, lots of photographs. And, yes, food.

Why would we want food to be a part of this? Well, isn't food a part of our lives? Isn't food reality? Don't we deal with food every day? Don't we have to eat? Hellohhhhh! Of course we had food.

This is about activity. This is about belonging. This is not about food.

I wasn't out to create a freak show, some special world for all of us "special" people to step into. That's not reality. The point of this entire program was to function in the real world, to climb out of that place of ill health and unhappiness and rejoin the real world.

Do people bring food to a party in the real world? Yes, they do. But what do we bring? We bring healthy food choices. Does that mean we can't bring a cake? Of course we can bring a cake, but maybe it's a fat-free angel food cake with fresh strawberries instead of a double chocolate New York cheesecake. And maybe we eat one piece instead of three.

Yes, we bring a vegetable tray, but is there never a bag of chips? Yes, there are chips, but instead of wolfing down a whole bag by yourself, you have just a few, you enjoy the taste. You're exercising a little control, and it's easier to do it there than anywhere else because you're surrounded by friends who are facing and doing the exact same thing.

At each one of these gatherings, I'd give out prizes and

awards, all honoring each member's effort and achievement during the previous three months. Recognition. Tons of recognition, regardless of the inches lost. It doesn't matter what you reward someone for, you just simply want to get them up and have people clapping for them, tossing confetti on them. Do you have any idea what it is like for people who have been isolated and alone for so long to step up and have a crown put on their head, to have a crowd of friends hooting and whistling and cheering for them as they parade around the room?

It's phenomenal. And a lot of them didn't want to do it at first. It was so hard for them. These are people who have been shrinking back all their lives, who don't want to stand out. They don't wear loud clothes. They don't wear bright colors. Some of them have a hard time even coming out of their house.

But they came out for this. And they liked it. They *loved* it.

Everyone got prizes, but there were winners and losers as well. Only one person could get the award for having lost the most inches. Only one winner. Did that make everyone else losers? Was it dangerous to have competition? Again, the answer is absolutely not. This was all about dealing with the real world, not being isolated in a little freak box. Is there competition in the real world? Is winning and losing and competing bad if it's handled and defined in a positive overall context? I don't think so.

There is competition in the real world. There are mirrors. There are ugly people who get in your face, and there are good people who are there to support you. That's reality. That's life. Sometimes you win, sometimes you lose. So do you avoid playing the game because you might not win? How real is that? How healthy is it?

My aim was to provide a safe environment for my students to measure their progress and to feel successful simply for staying the course, for simply continuing to try. And I applied the same principle of constant reward and reinforcement to another aspect of my program.

Behavior modification is what it was. I wanted to figure out a positive, healthy, doable way to begin tracking the behavioral habits — not just eating, because I didn't want this to be just about food — that were such a problem for so many of us, including me. The approach I came up with became one of the pinnacles of my program.

Along with the chart I kept in the classroom on which we recorded our inches-lost measurements, I made a list of behavioral habits, both good and bad. They ranged from drinking water to eating junk food, from daytime snacks to late-night feasting. Any habit I could think of, I put up on that chart, good ones as well as bad: having one night for yourself per week, or one hour for yourself per day; getting activity into your life in some way, shape or form; realizing that success begins with simply attempting to become aware of how you are living your life, of what you are doing with yourself and your body, both healthy and unhealthy. That's the incredibly important first step: awareness. Not judging or condemning. Not hypervigilant tension. I'm talking about an awareness couched in a cushion of gentleness and acceptance. The pursuit of a healthy body is not, and never should have been, about beating ourselves up. If there's one thing we should have learned by now, it's the futility of coming at this thing from that angle. Self-acceptance and self-love — that's the soil in which the seeds of a healthy transformation can truly take root and grow.

I preached that message — shared it and tried to show it — again and again with my classes. With that attitude established — that this is a positive thing, a growth thing, that it's not about punishment — each student then either chose one of those habits or came up with one of their own, and that became their focal point for the next ninety days. They may have had — and in most cases, did have — a lot more than one habit to deal with, but the key here was to focus on just one.

And with that one habit, the approach was to trim it down a little bit at a time, piece by piece, in tiny increments (in the case of bad habits), rather than trying to tackle it whole and just cut it out in one fell swoop. Or to build it up (in the case of good habits). How many times had we tried to do that? And how many times had it not worked?

Take the example of second helpings. There were more than a few people in my classes — including me — who would have as many as five helpings at a meal, on a regular basis. *Five.*

What that person would do is aim first at cutting back to four helpings over the course of, say, a couple of weeks. Nice and easy.

Then, when they're used to four, try getting down to three, again over a period of weeks. No rush. But constant awareness. Very important. We each have our own copy of our chart tacked up on the fridge at home. We keep a card to carry around with us during the day. All to remind us of that habit.

And eventually, after a couple of months, those five helpings are a memory, and we're having just seconds now, the way a "normal" person eats. And now maybe it's time to move on to another habit.

Constant awareness. Always making the attempt to keep "this" front and center, whatever "this" is for you, whether it's a healthy habit to nurture or a not-so-great habit to get rid of. Maybe it's a mind-set to work on. Maybe you aren't ready to actually work on it yet but you're in position to begin thinking about it. Awareness itself is an act, a step, a beginning, a movement in the right direction. Awareness itself is absolutely a form of success. Don't doubt that. Don't deny it. Let me tell you, denial can be a devil. Denial never did anyone any good. Awareness is quite the opposite of denial. Awareness is seeing something for what it is, and in this case it is seeing yourself for what you are and giving yourself credit not just for what you're doing but for how you're thinking, how you're feeling. It's recognizing that simply turning in the right direction, even before you actually begin moving, is an achievement in itself. Give yourself credit. Don't deny yourself what you deserve. Know that what you're doing is a good thing, and it can only lead to more good things. Reward yourself. Be honest with yourself, and be merciful as well.

Is there a challenge in front of you, a problem that seems so enormous, so big you can't get your arms around it, so large you can't imagine even beginning to tackle it? Break it apart, cut it down into doable pieces. Give yourself the room and the time to take on those pieces. One step at a time. Now we're getting somewhere. Now that tastes like success, rather than the quick-fix, take-it-all-on, change-everything-at-once approach we've all tried so many times — a guaranteed recipe for frustration and failure.

The key to this behavioral aspect of my program was the same as the key to our workouts, which was the same as the key to the measurements and the parties and the prizes, and that is that trying is succeeding.

Trying is succeeding.

Say it again.

TRYING IS SUCCEEDING.

I say that to myself every day, as many times as I can make myself aware to say it (there's that constant awareness thing again). An example occurred not so long ago, when my in-laws came to New York City to visit for the first time. The traditional tourist thing to do is visit the Statue of Liberty, so of course that's what we did. We went early one morning, riding over with a group of Statue employees before the actual opening time (my husband's Coastie status got us that "in"), so we had the place virtually to ourselves.

Once at the base of the Liberty Lady herself, I saw there was an elevator and a set of stairs with a big sign saying the only way to the top of the crown was the stairs. The elevator didn't go there.

In the quietness and vastness of this special place, I flashed back to all the times I had missed out on "trips to the top." Like a day at the beach, and everyone hikes to the top of a huge sand dune, and what would I do? Wasn't I dying to go up there with them? But knowing that I'd drop dead halfway up, I'd wave them on and stay at the bottom and watch, telling them I didn't want to go up the dune. Didn't want to go up the dune? Of course I wanted to go up there. But I couldn't do it, or I felt I couldn't do it, and so I simply pretended I didn't want to.

The same with swimming. I love the water. But when everyone else was suited up and diving into the lake or the pool or the ocean, I'd stay on the sand, in the lounge chair, out of the water, saying I did not like to swim, not admitting as a youngster that I was mortified that I probably didn't have the stamina to pass that swim test, or as an adult that I was ashamed of exposing myself as some sort of huge sea creature.

So I just stayed away. So many active, energetic, fun things in life, things that spoke directly to my own active, energetic, fun soul — I dodged them right and left, missing out on so much of life because of the combination of my physical condition and my terrible self-image.

I thought of all that as I looked up at that sign. All the coulda-woulda-shouldas of my past flashed before me, all the copouts and the waving away and the not trying. And I said to myself, Not this time! My in-laws stepped into that elevator, and I told them I'd meet them back at the bottom. They looked at me as if I was out of my mind, but the doors closed before they could say anything.

And so we began climbing, I and Jeremy, my younger son. I had one thing on my mind — the top of that crown. Step by step we went up, a year's worth of steps — 364, to be exact. Toward the top, Jeremy got frightened and back down he went. So it was me alone at the end, and I can't describe the euphoria I felt as I stepped into that crown, peered out those windows at the harbor below, the skyline, the horizon in all directions. I was literally and emotionally on top of the world!

I did not miss out on this one. That's what I told myself as I gazed out at that magnificent view. I was soaking wet with sweat. I mean, this was one heck of a workout. I felt so proud I could have burst — and Lady Liberty would have exploded right along with me. I just about floated down those steps, I was so filled with great feelings. When I got down to the base of the statue, there was the rest of the family to greet me, not with cheers or congratulations . . . but with the camera I'd forgotten to carry up with me.

The pictures! I forgot to get pictures. I looked over at Keith, and in that unmistakable, nonverbal way spouses can communicate with just a glance, he gave me a "No way am I climbing those steps with you." My mother-in-law looked at me, wringing wet, and said, "Well, Dee, you certainly can't go back up there."

Can't? Hmmmmmm. Wouldn't it be interesting if I did? That's what I thought as I shielded the morning sun from my eyes and gazed up at Lady Liberty's crown. Maybe Keith's mom was right. Maybe I couldn't make it. But I could try.

So back up those stairs I went, camera in hand. And I made it all the way. As I clicked off that roll of film, I was so elated I began to cry. I owned fitness. In spite of the size and shape I was, I was *fit*.

It's amazing those pictures came out focused. But they did, and when I got them back and was able to share that view with my family, who couldn't make it up to the top for much the same reasons I had stayed away from challenges before — that was as good as any gold medal for me.

To believe you can do something you never thought you could do before can seem like such a small step. To believe that the simple act of trying, whether you actually do it or not, is success in itself, is not easy for people who are used to nothing but failure and feeling like failures.

But it works. Believe me, it works. And it was working every day in that studio at Gigi's. This wasn't just a lot of hocus-pocus. This wasn't smoke and mirrors. That was real sweat happening in that room. That was real knowledge being shared and absorbed in those postworkout "class" sessions. Those were real inches lost on those charts. Those were real habits being changed.

And the joy swelling out of the faces of the students and their families and their friends at every one of our ninety-day Celebrations, that was real, too.

Chapter

10

Hanging with the Bad Boys

B y the beginning of 1993, my program was going great
guns. More than two hundred women and men were
enrolled, including a half dozen or so who were working with me to become instructors themselves, soaking up
the approach and sensitivity I'd tried to develop to effectively work with people whose instinct is to hide or quit
when the word "exercise" comes up.

As for myself, I was in tremendous physical condition
despite the fact that I still weighed well over two hundred.
Keep in mind that I had weighed over three hundred when
I first stepped through Gigi's door four years earlier.

The bottom line in terms of my weight was that as the
program grew, as classes were added, I was teaching more —
I was teaching them all. First three, then four, then six, and
finally ten. I wasn't paying any attention to my weight. I
was just having a blast, day in and day out. I knew I was

feeling fit, thanks to my constant activity and to my newly developed relationship with food. I now saw food primarily as fuel. I had dived into learning what makes the body work, into physiology and anatomy, and I was applying to myself and to my students as much as I could of what I was learning. Most important, I was practicing everything I preached, including ignoring the scales. What weight I lost was a byproduct I didn't even notice — a byproduct of my entire lifestyle.

I had become immersed in the subculture of fitness, even to the point of my wardrobe, which now included a glittery, electric-blue spandex bodysuit, size 2X. I got it at Wal-Mart.

Me in spandex. I never thought I'd see the day. To me, spandex had always been something all these little girls trotted around in, showing off their bodies, thinking they were such hot stuff. Well, guess what? When I finally put it on, I found out it has a function. You wear spandex because you can move in it, and because when you sweat — I mean, really sweat — you can still move. Wow, Dee, what a revelation! There's a purpose for these things. And all this time I thought they were just to look good and show off and be shiny.

Something else I had always thought was that physical competition, athletic tests of endurance or skill, were in another universe from mine, a world apart from the one in which I lived. Me taking part in a sport? I couldn't even climb a flight of stairs. Or, rather, I couldn't imagine climbing a flight of stairs. Or walking to the top of a sand dune to see the splendor of a sunset. Or hiking down a valley to witness the beauty of a waterfall. Or climbing into a rowboat for a ride down a river. These were things I'd missed out on my entire life because I was too embarrassed, too ashamed and simply too *afraid* to put my body to any kind of test, especially in full view of other people. Of course I never admitted I was afraid or ashamed. No, the family would be begging me to come on, Mom, let's do this, or let's do that, and every time I'd say, You guys go ahead, I'll stay here. Every time.

I spent a lifetime of never getting to do anything because I didn't feel I could. I didn't feel I should. I didn't feel I *deserved* it. Do you know what I'm talking about? Does this sound familiar? You go out for a day on the river, it's ninety degrees, it's sweltering, and you're fully clothed. You're ready for a hike in the Rockies!

And everyone's climbing into canoes, and you're looking at this thing and saying to yourself, No way. I put one foot in that sucker, and it's going down. And they're all gonna know it's me that did it.

So I'd just wave them on, say go ahead without me, as if I didn't want to ride in that canoe, as if I didn't want to see that sunset, as if I didn't want to feel the spray from that waterfall.

Who was I fooling? Who are you fooling?

Well, let me tell you, by the time I was suiting up in spandex, there was no holding me back anymore. I knew by then that this whole out-of-shape thing has nothing to do with size, with medical background, with where you start, with how old or young you are, with whether you're pink, purple, or green, male or female. I knew by then that this is not about boundaries, that fitness is for everybody, just like life is.

But you know what? You've got to believe it to achieve it. I'll say it again. You've got to *believe* it to *achieve* it. If you don't believe you deserve to be healthy, to be alive, to have fun in this world in an active, participatory sense, then you won't. You won't have what it takes to get there, to do it, to be it, if you don't believe it. And you won't believe it if you don't think you deserve it. Before and above anything else in this world, you have to convince yourself that you deserve what you want. Otherwise you'll be beaten before you begin. I've been there. I know what that feels like. You do, too.

So how do you take that first step? You do it by acting *as if*. You do it by stepping beyond the misconceptions, the stereotypes and labels and prejudices we all face. You do it by believing in yourself, by telling yourself you deserve this, and then by acting as if you can do and be whatever you choose. Set your sights on that goal, whatever it is, then commit yourself totally to that reality. Approach it as if it is absolutely, unquestionably true. And it will become true.

Believe it, then achieve it. Take those resolutions that in the past have been dropped by the wayside like so much litter and watch them turn into commitments. Then watch those commitments turn into lifestyle, life-enhancing habits. And watch how your life changes. You're going to live longer. You're going to live better. And you're going to find more potential and achieve more goals than you ever dreamed.

Let me tell you a story, something that happened to me that spring of 1993. Something that tells you all about goals, and believing, and achieving. I heard about a bike race coming up in Lake Charles. That's right. A bike race.

Now, you're talking about somebody who had never competed in an athletic event in her life. Are you kidding me? Walking from my car to the front door of the mall was an athletic event for me.

But things were changing now. My life was changing. My body had changed. I'd been losing inches, I'd lost some pounds, I had a full head of steam with my classes, and, I don't know, maybe it was just time to take this step, this big, big step, but when I heard about this big race coming up in a couple of months, something in my head said, Do it.

So I did. They had a sixty-miler, a thirty-miler, and a ten-miler. I set my sights on the thirty. I told myself that if I practiced and could get up to thirty miles, regardless of my time, then I'd try to go forty. And if I could go forty miles in practice, then I could finish a thirty-mile race. That was my mind-set.

So I began training. Every day I thought, "I can't believe I'm going to do this." It was like a game I was playing with myself, like a half-hearted attempt just to see how badly I'd do. We've all got our little brain games we have to play when those demons of self-doubt start beating their wings around us, and this was my game, taking this thing dead seriously on the one hand but at the same time treating it like a lark, an adventure.

Well, I got up to forty miles. I didn't worry about the time at all. I didn't worry about how long it took me. Maybe it'd take me a day and a half, I didn't care. I mean, my backside cared a little bit. I mean, sitting on that teeny little bike seat for that amount of time can be very detrimental to your sense of well-being . . .

In any event, I kept going, and when I got up to forty-five miles, I said to myself, By God, I'm gonna do this race!

The day came, a terrible, terrible day. Dark, windy, storm clouds rolling overhead, rain coming down in sheets. The weather was so bad they canceled the sixty-miler. They kept the thirty and the ten, so the thirty-miler was filled with all these people who had been planning to do the sixty, these Tour de France specimens. A lot of the thirty-mile crowd was dropping down to the ten. But not me, babe. I told myself I'd worked my bazooka off for this thirty-mile ride and I was doing the thirty miles. I didn't care if it was raining and I had to wear plastic bags all over my body and look like a geek on that bike. I was doing it.

So I climbed on my bicycle, and the thing started, and everyone took off, and there I was, in the lead pack, right out front. Now for me, being out there in the lead pack, hanging with the bad boys, well, you can imagine what a mind-blower that was. I mean, Whoa, quit it!

Well, then the lead pack broke into two groups, and now I was in the second lead pack. I'm not in the first lead pack anymore, so I break it down in my head and tell myself I'm in the second lead pack. Whatever works, right?

The rain was really coming down now, and I was really kicking it, hanging with that second lead pack, and we came up on a railroad crossing, and as I went across, my wheels hit those wet, slick rails . . .

And I lost it.

My bike went skidding in one direction, and I went flying in the other. I hydroplaned about fifteen feet, tore the living daylights out of the left side of my body, ripped my brand-new biking pants. Broke two knuckles in my right hand. Blood everywhere.

I'm lying there in the middle of the road, the second-lead pack out of view and nobody behind me, and I'm stretched out on my back looking up at the sky and thinking, "Okay, God. What's the plan here?"

I mean, this was one of those moments, you know? What was I supposed to do? I wasn't even thinking about how my body hurt — I thought about that plenty later. But at that moment all I could think about was how long and how hard I'd trained for this thing. I looked over at my bike, bent up in a ditch like something somebody had thrown out, and I told myself, If that thing still works, I'm getting back ON that sucker.

And I did.

And I finished that race. I never even stopped at any of the break points. And you know what else? I wasn't even the last one across that finish line.

That was an incredible experience for me. That was the first time in my life that I got even just a little taste of what physical competition — real, hard-nosed, top-elite competition — is like. That was my first taste of what actual athletes go through, in terms of training and competing and committing themselves to staying the course no matter what. I'd never felt that kind of high before, not in a physical sense. I knew how to compete, and I'd achieved plenty using my mind, in school and in the workplace. But never had I put my body through something like this. Never had I felt the personal satisfaction, the sense of achievement I felt that day.

And it had nothing to do with competing against anyone else. The race, the bikers all around me, that was just the setting. It had everything to do with challenging myself, committing to the hard, hard work of training, and then facing, sticking with, and surmounting the walls I ran into during that thirty-mile race. That's when I got my first sense of what they mean when they say, There *is* no finish line. Not in the big picture. Life is filled with one challenge after another, one tiny finish line after another, and the sweetness is not in the winning or losing but in the satisfaction of staying with it, of trying, of reaching for one rung in the ladder after another.

Of course I'm not just talking about thirty-mile races. I'm talking about maybe turning off the TV and getting up and going for a walk around the block. I'm talking about maybe taking the stairs up to that second-floor office rather than riding the elevator. I'm talking about parking at the back of the lot rather than at the front and walking that extra distance to the mall. I'm talking about maybe reaching for an apple here and there instead of a bag of potato chips.

Steps on the ladder, one rung after another.

It was about the time of that bike race that I got my first shot at teaching a regular class, a room full of Gigi's regulars, well-oiled aerobic machines straight out of a fitness video. I'd talked for some time to Gigi about trying this, just to see how it could go, just to test my own limits, and she was not exactly excited. "I don't mean to hurt your feelings," she told me, "but I wonder if these people would want you to teach them?" They might be uncomfortable, even offended. Gigi was careful about how she said it, but that's what she was telling me. Which, of course, made me only more determined to do it.

My chance came when one of Gigi's instructors called one afternoon from Houston, where she was held up at the airport. She wouldn't be able to make it back to teach that night's class. Gigi was already gone for the day. No one was available to fill in — no one but me.

I've got to admit I wasn't sure if I wanted to do it. I had my doubts. I mean, this was a reality I hadn't stepped into. The big thong thing. These men and women with their incredible bodies. I was super confident with everything I'd already done and could do, with the program I'd built and what I'd proved to myself and my students. I knew I had all the tools to teach anyone, even Gigi's best. But I hadn't actually *done* it. I was still on the outside looking in when it came to them, that incredible 5:30 afternoon class. They were still like gods and goddesses to me.

There were fifty people in that class, the largest Gigi had — about the same number as my largest. I was intimidated, nervous, practically petrified, if you want to know the truth. I had no idea whether I might be getting in over my head here. Minutes before class time that day, I stood out in the hall, suited up in my spandex, still deciding. The room was filling up with stretching, pacing aerobic animals, only a couple of whom were even aware of what was going on. One of them, a woman named Debby, came out and walked over to me.

"Shoot, Dee," she said, "you can do this. We know how to high-impact. We'll high-impact, you low. Come on, let's go."

She was great. That's all I needed.

I stepped in and everyone looked up.

"Hi, y'all," I said. "Some of you know me, some might not. My name's Dee, and I teach VVV."

Vim, Vigor and Vital — that's what my program was called at the time.

"Pam's not going to be here tonight," I continued, "so I'll be doing it, if everybody feels okay about that."

Well, one young lady did not feel okay about it. Thin, sleek, with "prissy girl" written all over every gesture she made, she walked up to me and said, "I don't mean to be rude, but you're just too big. You can't possibly provide me with a good workout." And she walked out.

Talk about your reality check. I was devastated. You only *think* you're good, I thought to myself. You're really just a fat piece of garbage. That's what was racing through my head. Oh no, I thought, who am I trying to kid?

But then another woman — one of the studio's real mainstay students; small but muscular, dark shoulder-length hair, with the cardiovascular system of a horse — came right over and said, "It's all right, Dee. Just do it. Let's go. We're ready." Then she went back to her spot.

And so I did. I just did it. Cued the music, stepped up . . . and rocked . . . their . . . world.

I mean, we cooked. They knew the patterns, they knew the drill, and they were right with me. A hundred and fifty-seven beats per minute, the rhythm was thumping. If they went high where I couldn't, then I stayed low, still leading, still on top of it, pushing them, pumping them, cueing, shifting, sliding into the conditioning segment, three sets of fifteen, with the weights. Then the steps, on the incline, and if I couldn't stay up on the step, I kept flat on the floor, still moving, guiding, leading them, doing it.

Did *I* get an incredible workout? I'm not supposed to get an incredible workout. I'm not there to get a workout for me. I'm there to provide a safe, effective workout for them. I'm not there to show what I can do, to strut my stuff and look at myself in the mirror and be Miss Aerobic America. I'm there to motivate them. This is their workout, not mine.

And I gave them a workout. When it was done, they were all over me.

"Dee, that was fantastic."

"Dee, that was great."

"Dee, that kicked ass!"

What a blast. Any sense that I might still be separated from the real deal vanished that night. From that point on, I was not only an aerobics instructor who taught this special program. I was an aerobics instructor, period.

My own students were beginning to make the same kind of transition, several of them "graduating," in a sense, from my program and moving on their own into one of the higher-impact classes. That was one of the most incredible things for me to watch, to see some of my students, after a year or two in the program, go over to the hardbody class. They'd come back to me and say, "Dee, oh Dee, we miss you. Don't be mad." Don't be mad? That's what this is all about, I'd tell them. Don't ever apologize for getting fit enough to go out there and kick butt.

By now, it was beginning to become clear that Gigi and I were approaching a parting of the ways. The club simply wasn't big enough for both of us. I had become a local celebrity of sorts, drawing lots of attention from the Lake Charles newspapers and television stations. Who wouldn't start to get uncomfortable about that? I understood the tension that was beginning to develop between Gigi and me. I could never thank her enough for her support, her expertise, the guidance she gave me in my evolution from unfit medical nightmare to fitness instructor. Gigi took a chance on me and my ideas when I doubt others would have. Think about it. Who would — who will — take a chance on you?

Still and all, by the summer of 1993, it was pretty clear to me that things were coming toward a head, that it was time to be looking to leave. Where to go was another question. I was still a Coast Guard wife, still tied to Keith's career. And I had little knowledge of the fitness industry as a business, of how to start and run my own operation, rather than working for someone else. I was learning, though. The summer before, I had attended a regional fitness conference in Dallas, where I had floated some of my ideas and innovations for the first time among industry insiders, testing the waters to possibly branch out on my own.

I've got to admit I really had some balls to do that. I walked right into that convention without a shred of self-doubt, started passing out these packets explaining my program, cornering people and telling them what I had here, that I had something that worked, that was different, that people needed to know about, that I needed to share.

That Texas deal was a good experience, but it was much smaller than the worldwide fitness industry convention that was approaching the following summer in, of all places, New Orleans. My trip to Dallas had been like a scouting expedition. By the time the New Orleans event arrived, I was ready to launch a full-scale attack.

The site was the city's convention center, which, on this muggy week in July, had been transformed into a Valhalla of exercise. More than four thousand men and women, representatives from every facet of the fitness industry around the globe, had gathered under that domed roof to sell, buy, and promote the latest lines of health and exercise products and programs.

Like any such convention, the place was a carnival-like ocean of booths, workshops, panel discussions, speeches, demonstrations, and displays meant to dazzle and lure the throngs roaming the aisles and hallways. Naturally, as ever, I stuck out like an apple in a bowl of cherries.

It was the same old drill. Glares, stares, people treating me like a cute little pet, others looking at me as if I were diseased. But that was fine. I was there with a purpose — to spread the word about my program and to pick up whatever I could find that I might be able to use. I was there to learn as much as anything else.

And I did. I spent that entire week working those halls, handing out pamphlets and brochures and picking the brains of anyone who would speak to me. By the time I sat down at the banquet that marked the end of the event, I knew I'd done all I could. I listened to the master of ceremonies announce that the next year's gathering would be held in Las Vegas. Then I watched as a representative from the Nike Corporation stepped up to the microphone to make an announcement of his own. Nike, he said, was launching an annual competition with a hefty award — a

$25,000 grant, a product-endorsement contract, and a perpetual trophy — to encourage and reward the development of innovative programs in the industry.

My jaw dropped. I felt this man was speaking directly to me. Four thousand people in this room, and here's little chubby Dee, sitting there and saying to myself, "I'm going to win this thing."

Of course as soon as I thought that, I said to myself, "No, no, no. You *want* to win it." That was that old fear of failure kicking in, that caution about setting myself up for disappointment. But it didn't last more than an instant.

"No," I corrected myself again, "I mean I'm *going* to win this award. This was made for me."

That's how I felt when I left that conference that night. No doubt in my mind. Everything I'd done, everything I was about, was meant for this.

And with that, I loaded my boys and our luggage into the family Dodge and pointed it north to join Keith at his new job. That's right. After five years in Louisiana, the Coast Guard had decided that it was time for the Hakalas to move again. And this time we were being transferred to a billet stranger than anything I could have imagined.

This time we were moving to New York City.

11

On the Island

The timing of that move to New York was as if destiny were kicking in, cooperating in a way I could never have dreamed of. I knew the time had come for the next step in my new career — taking my program solo, out from under the umbrella of someone else's operation. I had no idea, however, where or when or how I might make that move.

Until Uncle Sam made it for me. When Keith was assigned to the Coast Guard's national base of operations at Governors Island, New York, that summer of 1993, my students at Gigi's were heartbroken, but they were left in good hands. I had worked hard at preparing some of them to become instructors themselves. It was now left to them to carry on the work I'd begun.

Meanwhile, it was left to me to move my family and myself into a home unlike any I had known before. Talk about a *trip*. It was surreal. One day we're living in the heart of Cajun country, the swamps of Louisiana, the next we're on this *island*, right there at the mouth of the Hudson and the East Rivers, moving into an apartment literally in the shadow of the Manhattan skyline and the Brooklyn Bridge, close enough to throw a rock at the World Trade Center. I woke up that first morning, opened my bedroom blinds, and I was looking straight at the blessed Statue of Liberty. Incredible.

Governors Island was literally a world unto itself, a self-contained community, a speck of water-bound land roughly two and a half miles in circumference, with about two thousand inhabitants — Coast Guard personnel and their families. It had its own school, its own grocery store, its own base newspaper, movie theater, bowling alley, swimming pool, gymnasium, soccer and baseball fields — even a golf course. The canyons of Wall Street were a mere fifteen-minute ferry ride away, and those free military ferries ran nonstop from dawn until midnight. But a person living on Governors Island might never set foot on one of those ferries and still enjoy everything he — or she — needed right there on the island.

Everything, that is, except a full-fledged fitness center.

Talk about coming into a place with a need. I couldn't believe it. The largest Coast Guard base in the world, and they basically had nothing. Not that they weren't trying, but it just wasn't a priority, and they really didn't know what they were doing. What they called a fitness center was nothing more than a room with a bunch of equipment in it, some of it pretty antiquated, most of it not used at all. They had an aerobics class going, with volunteer instructors, which was *something*. But anyone interested in a serious, high-quality, professional workout had to take a ferry into the city and go to one of the Vic Tanny or Bally's or Jazzercise studios there. If you didn't want to do that, if you didn't want to ferry over and have to deal with the subways and the taxis and the tall buildings in a single bound, then you were stuck. There was nothing for you on Governors Island.

Which actually made it a godsend for me, a perfect place to try launching my program, to take it solo for the first time. That was the challenge I was facing before I even found out we were leaving Louisiana. Could I do this on my own? I would have wound up trying it wherever we might have moved, but it would have been tougher out there in the world of strip malls and shopping centers and the yellow pages full of hundreds of aerobics studios. Out there I would have been a voice in the wilderness, at least at first. But here I was literally on an island, the only game in town. It was like having my own little laboratory.

Not that it would be easy getting started. This was, after all, a military base, with all the rigidity and bureaucracy that that entails. Anyone who's ever lived the military life knows what I'm talking about. They don't like change in the military. Change is hard in any large institution, but the military is in a class by itself when it comes to rules, regulations, tradition. If you try to change, try to introduce anything that's new, you're going to face resistance and red tape every step of the way, just a maze of questions and paperwork and procedure.

That's exactly what I ran into when I first floated my program to the island's powers-that-be. I went and talked to the base sports director and he said, No way, it's not going to happen. It's *never* going to happen, he said. Other people had tried to set up something permanent such as I was suggesting, and it never lasted, he said. People leave. They're transferred. They quit. Whatever. It won't work. It's *never* worked.

Well, that's the wrong thing to say to me. Tell me no, and I'm going to come back at you even harder, especially when it comes to fitness.

In this case, I decided to go straight to the top. I wrote a letter to the base commander, explaining my background, my credentials, my program, the need I saw on the island and how I planned to answer that need. And that got me a meeting with the big honcho, the top dog, the commander of the U.S. Coast Guard Support Center, Governors Island, New York. He was camped behind the hugest desk I'd ever seen, wearing his crisp dress blues, flags behind him, plaques all over the walls, all that good military stuff. It could have been pretty intimidating if I weren't so used to that scene. But I was; I'd seen more commanding officers' digs during Keith's career than I could count. I was certainly respectful, but I wasn't there to salute. I was there to show this man what I had to offer his men and their families. I laid out everything, very detailed, very professional. I told him what they had going was fine, but they needed something more formalized, more structured. I gave him my résumé and told him I'd like to start an aerobics program that would be for everyone on that island — men, women, the unconditioned, the supertoned athlete — *everyone*. Hey, this place was and always had been, in essence, a fort. What better place for a warrior like me, right?

Well, that's not the way the CO saw it. You know what

he saw? He saw an enlisted man's wife. An aggressive enlisted man's wife. An *overweight* assertive enlisted man's
wife. That was it. That was all. Period.

Another "No." So I tried a different tack. I put together
a survey and went house to house, apartment to apartment, covering the entire island, knocking on the doors of
officers and enlisted men alike, collecting data ranging
from what people were willing to pay to how the issue of
child care might be handled.

The response was overwhelming. Now I had numbers.
Not only that, but I had names. A month later I was back
at the base headquarters, this time for a dressing-down
from the island's comptroller. When he heard what I was
doing, he yanked my butt in so fast it would make your
head spin. He said, "You can't do surveys without government approval, blah, blah, blah."

I said, "Whatever." I'd never lived on a base before. I
understood about the regulations. But I told him what I'd
told the commander. I want *fitness* in this place, I said. You
need this. This resistance you're putting up is ridiculous.
Let's do it. Then I gave him a detailed proposal about how
we could do it so it would be cost effective, how the base
would get its percentage, et cetera. And we came up with a
contract. I signed it at the start of October, and by the end
of that month, I had my first class going.

I did it the same way I'd done it in Lake Charles, using
flyers to lure students, that and an ad in the base newspaper. Fifteen men and women showed up for my first class,
on a Monday morning, in a third-floor room of one of the
base's old brick buildings, a room also used for children's
dance classes. Cracked linoleum-tile floor. Paint peeling

around the windows. This was an old building. An old, old building. How old? Half the buildings on the island were designated historical sites. This place had been settled for over 350 years. Ben Franklin slept here. So did George Washington. Wilbur Wright showed off his new flying machine here in 1909, taking off from Governors Island for a spin around the Statue of Liberty. I mean, this place had some *age* on it.

Which didn't mean it was necessarily in great shape. In fact, "historical" is often just another word for run-down and falling apart. That was certainly true in the case of my classroom. But I didn't care. I had what I needed, and I went at it with the same fire that had burned in me for the previous four years.

I'd proved at Gigi's that I could teach both specialized students with physical limitations *and* top-conditioned athletes. Here, I faced the challenge of applying my program to that same range of students not in separate settings, but in the same room at the same time.

And it worked. We did it all. Keeping the diary logs, charting the behaviors, bringing in the educational aspect, the experts, having the contests and Celebrations, giving out the awards. The foundation in the workout room itself remained the same, reaching out, identifying and tailoring the routines to the specific needs of each student. But there were students in there who had no specific needs, athletes and hardbodies doing the workouts right alongside the people with weight problems and the diabetics, and *everybody* got what they needed. Everyone came away from each class with the benefit of a safe, thorough aerobic workout.

Actually, the biggest challenge I faced was not the

range of my students' physical limitations, but the range of their military rank. There is no place in America more stratified and class-conscious than a military base. The lines drawn between officers and enlisted men — and their wives and families — are amazing.

Right off the bat I announced that there was going to be none of that in this room. The prejudices, the barriers, the tit-for-tat — all that stripes-and-bars stuff was staying outside. This was about fitness, I said, and fitness doesn't give a damn about your rank. How well your heart beats, how efficiently your blood pumps, how strong your muscles are — those things have nothing to do with whether you're an admiral or a chief, a commander's wife or a seaman's daughter. If you're wearing bars on your shoulders, I said, you'd better just take them off before you step through those doors, because they don't belong in this room. They did as I asked. Those bars and barriers really came down.

That first winter was hard, really hard. My classes quickly grew to the point where I needed a bigger workout room, and they gave me one, in the gymnasium of the island's elementary school. I was teaching five classes a week by then — one each night. But my equipment — the dozens of benches and risers my classes used during the course of each workout — remained stored in that third-floor room of the base's "MWR" (Morale, Welfare, and Recreation) building where we'd started out. The school gym was halfway across the island. So each afternoon, my routine began with a half dozen trips up and down those stairs, loading that equipment into my pickup truck, driving it across the island to the gym, and unloading it. Each evening, the routine was reversed as I hauled the stuff back to its storage place.

There were about thirty benches to load and unload. I'd take them four or five at a time. No elevator. Just the stairs. And then I had to load the risers. They took a couple more trips. It got to the point where it took longer to haul that stuff back and forth than it did to teach the classes. It was much more of a workout, I'll tell you that. I'd finish making a haul, and I'd be soaking wet from the sweat, sitting at the bottom of those steps to catch my breath, repeating to myelf over and over and over, like a chant, "*In the name of fitness. In the name of fitness. In the name of FITNESS!*"

The work itself was all good exercise, I could tell myself that, and it was true. But when the ice and the snow set in, that was bad. Some nights, just getting from the door out to the truck was like trekking through the tundra. I almost killed myself a couple of times, slipping on that ice.

I know I looked like a maniac, hauling this stuff around like that in the dead of winter. At one point the Command asked me why I didn't ask the students to help, let them carry their own equipment. I said, Absolutely not. They're paying for this class, I said. This was a full-service, professional program I was offering here. I wasn't about to ask people who were paying me for my services to help me do my job. Now and then some of my students did help. Keith and the boys pitched in, too. But most of the time it was just me, and that was fine.

By the spring of 1994, I was teaching fifteen classes a week. I had more than two hundred students enrolled, including several officers' wives who went to their husbands and, shall we say, urged them to provide better accommodations for my program.

Well, the next thing I knew, we had our own actual aerobics room. Building 400, Section G, on the second floor. Dark red bricks outside, high ceilings and windows in. They mounted mirrors on the walls. We painted it ourselves. And one of my students, a great gung-ho captain, pulled some strings and got $5,000 worth of specialized aerobic carpeting installed. By the end of that spring, we were good to go.

By then I had proved to myself, as well as to my students, that what I had to offer was truly something special, something unlike anything any of them — fit or unfit — had ever experienced. We were *doing* it, and it was *working*. Lives were being affected, changed for the better, right along with the bodies. There was a lot more than just inches being lost in that room. People were getting rid of pills, putting away medicine they'd been taking for years, because now they didn't need it anymore. Listen to what one of my earliest students on the island had to say in a letter she wrote in the spring of 1994 after six months in my program:

> *Greetings from Governors Island!*
>
> *First, let me introduce myself. My name is Debra Brand. I am a twenty-six-year-old female. I am a civil engineer working in Manhattan.*
>
> *While in high school, I was diagnosed with rheumatoid arthritis. During the four years I've been on Governors Island, my condition has worsened. In August of 1990 I was taking an anti-malarial drug and antiinflammatories. By August of 1993 I was taking chemotherapy (methotrexate — six 2.5 mg tablets weekly), steroids (Prednisone — two 5 mg tablets daily, with additional cortisone shots on an as-needed basis),*

and an anti-inflammatory called Relafen (two 500 mg tablets daily).

Since beginning aerobic classes with Dee in August of 1993, I have been able to reduce the prednisone from two tablets daily to only one, and I have reduced the chemotherapy tablets from six a week to five. I am hoping that by next winter I will be off the prednisone entirely and have lowered the chemotherapy medication even more.

As for my weight, in the last four years I had put on over twenty pounds, which for others may not seem to be a big deal, but it was for me (I gained ten pounds in 1993 alone). The extra weight gain had caused additional wear and tear on joints that were already afflicted with pain.

Since my initial measurement by Dee, I have lost over five and a half inches in my upper arms, chest, waist, hips, thighs, and calves. Along with the inches lost, I lost over ten pounds as well. Those inches and pounds lost are all due to my participation in Dee's class, and I mean participation!

Another of my Governors Island students, Diane Towers, shared her own story in a letter, also written that spring:

I am a thirty-two-year-old female who is overweight and in much need of some form of exercise. I have high blood pressure, high cholesterol, and hypothyroidism, all of which are heredity-related from my parents. At the time I first came to Dee Hakala's class, I had no energy, no self-esteem, and a doctor who was after me all

*the time to lose weight, lower my LDL, and increase
my HDL cholesterol.*

When I first met Dee, I could see she was one of us,
she had been there, and she was proof that overweight
people could exercise and keep up with a program.
Still, I wasn't sure I could do it. I'm not really into exercise. I can never keep up, and I feel like I'm wasting
my time. Once I joined a spa, but I could never keep
up with the classes and I hated the exercise machines,
so that was the end of that. Three hundred dollars
down the tubes.

The first day I came to Dee's class, I left early. I "had
something to do." She was using chairs that day, and I
thought to myself, "Exercising in chairs? How much
could you get out of that?" More than you can imagine,
but I didn't know that. The following week I stayed and
participated in the entire class. What a booster! Not
only could I keep up, but I was sweating, really having
a workout, and I didn't feel the next day like every
muscle in my body hurt. I decided this was for me.

As we were ready, Dee began increasing the times
per week we exercised and the length of each class. In
no time at all we were introduced to the "step." Imagine having enough energy to work on the step when
you are overweight. I used to watch my sister-in-law,
who is thin as a rail, on the step and knew I could
never do that. "Oh, my poor heart." I'd be so out of
breath. Now I not only can do it, but I really enjoy it.

If there's a central ingredient to Dee's program, it's
the fact that she modifies the exercise, whatever it is, for
you. In the first few months that I started exercising with

her, sometimes I would have problems with my lower legs; after not too long, they would go numb. (This was due to the hypothyroidism, which was not under control yet.) Dee modified the routine so we had more warm-up time, which really eased the numbing problem and helped me get through the rest of the class. In other words, with Dee's approach, you never miss out on something because you can't do it. She always has an adjustment or an alternative that you can do.

I've never exercised for more than a few weeks, but I have been going to Dee's classes for six months now. I have increased my HDL from 32 to 45, and needless to say, my doctor thinks this is great. Even though I haven't lost too many pounds, each time I visit my doctor, she can see how much better my body looks, how all the parts are much firmer and look nicer. Even my husband can notice.

All I can say is WOW!

Me, too. By the spring of '94, my students were hauling in their friends, making them come and be a part of this. It was going gangbusters, just as I thought it would, just as I knew it would. How could it not? Spring turned to summer, and early that June, as I was getting ready to leave my apartment one afternoon to head to the studio, my phone rang.

I had spent much of the previous winter putting together my pitch for that Nike prize. I had collected letters like the ones above from dozens of my students, in both Louisiana and New York. I had detailed the specifics of my program, describing each facet of the "New Face of Fitness" and explaining how my approach not only answered the needs of students with limitations but could also be applied to athletes who had none. I described how my instructors — many overweight like me, just as many in peak physical condition — were trained. A captain's wife, my friend Erin Bohner, pitched in with a computer and printer. Erin was great. And so wise. As I was finishing up the package, she said, "Dee, this is the best you can do. You know that, and you know that this program is perfect." Then she put both hands on my shoulders and said, "If you don't win, it won't be because you or your program aren't any good. It will be because the industry and society just aren't ready. People just aren't ready."

I knew what Erin was saying to me. I knew exactly what she meant. It would be very unlikely that the fitness industry would be ready for somebody my size representing their profession. Erin was being loving, but she was also being frank. She was giving me a big-time reality check, trying to prepare me for disappointment because she cared about me so much.

So, late that winter, as the ice and snow set in, I had put together and mailed off my package. Now it was summer. That award was the last thing on my mind as I grabbed the phone. I was in a hurry. I had a class to get to.

A woman was on the line. An unfamiliar voice, asking if this was Dee Hakala.

Somebody trying to sell something, that's what I thought. I was in a rush.

"Yeah, this is Dee." I said. "Who is this?"

"Well," said the woman, "I work for Nike."

12

Mount Olympus

thought it was a prank at first, some friend yanking my chain. Then I realized it was true, and I started stammering like a complete idiot.

"Really?"

"Really?"

"Really?"

That was all I kept saying.

I'd never won anything in my life except for a little bottle of Bonne Bell skin cream they gave away in a department store drawing back when I was living in Michigan. Now it was Nike, the first and last word in fitness, the top of freaking Mount Olympus, calling to tell me I'd won this thing. I mean, my mind was absolutely blown. A billion thoughts were flying through my brain, a billion questions, but all this woman wanted to know, all she kept asking me, was how I spelled my name. They needed to get it right on the trophy. Was it Dee with one *e* or two?

Who cares, I thought. Put an X on it. Gimme a G. Whatever! I mean, this is the biggest moment of my life and we're talking about how many *E*'s in Dee?

It turned out that a panel of industry experts assembled by the San Diego–based group IDEA (International Association of Fitness Professionals) had combed through more than eighty applications from across the country before choosing mine as the winner. The annual IDEA World Conference — the same convention I had attended in New Orleans the summer before — was scheduled for Las Vegas that month. I had already planned to attend, enrolling as a volunteer worker, manning a registration booth in return for a cut in my registration fee.

Now I'd be attending as a guest of honor. It's funny how things can change so fast. One minute I was a nobody, just a face in the crowd, and the next I was right up there with the fast-lane fitness crowd. Fitness industry representatives from more than sixty nations were there, more than four thousand business executives, salespeople, physicians, instructors, and athletes demonstrating every conceivable exercise device. Aerobic boxers, in-line skaters, dancers, people rope-skipping, doing water aerobics, flipping through the air on bicycles — there were stages all over the place, with presentations, demonstrations, classes, and lectures going on all day long, every day for a week. An amazing scene, like a combination expo/circus. Of course, this was Las Vegas.

All that week, people I had never met slipped me their

business cards. Gym managers asked me how to get a franchise, told me my program was like nothing they'd ever heard of before. It was pretty amazing.

The final night of the convention, all four thousand attendees gathered for a banquet and awards ceremony. Men in black tie, women in sequined gowns. I swear, it was like the Academy Awards. Entertainment ranged from rappers and hip-hop dancers to in-line skaters and mountain bike acrobats. A parade of award winners followed, each of them stepping up to the stage to receive a plaque or a trophy. One was the creator of a tumbling program for inner-city kids in Chicago. Another was a woman with multiple sclerosis who had completed six straight New York City marathons.

Finally, a Nike vice president stepped to the podium to present the evening's final honor, Nike's Fitness Innovation Award. The four finalists were introduced, then the winner was announced.

I have a videotape of that moment, and it's still unreal to watch myself, wearing a floor-length gown with a rainbow-colored sequined jacket, my hair cut shoulder length and full, walking toward that stage amid a standing ovation, flashing a thumbs-up to the crowd and reaching out to grip this huge, three-foot-high granite, marble, crystal, and brass obelisk Nike had created as its trophy for this award. All I could think about as I climbed the steps to that stage was making sure I did whatever it took not to fall down! I'd watched one of the previous award winners that night stumble on those steps. I could see it happening to me. "Lord," I prayed as I walked toward that stage, the people applauding all around me, "please don't let me trip and fall and have my dress blow up over my head and my whole backside show for the world to see. Amen. Thank You."

You know how they say your life passes before your eyes when you're just about to die? Well, I'll tell you, my life did pass before my eyes as I stood on that stage, looking out on that ocean of people, all applauding. I thought about my dad, my family, and our life growing up, the years I lived by myself, so alone, the hopelessness, the emptiness I felt for so long. And then the way out that I'd finally found, the way up, the people I'd helped and who had helped *me* more than they could ever know, the way my life was continuing to change every day, changes that were never going to stop, not anymore, because there's no stopping anymore when you're really alive — truly, healthily alive.

I'd stopped so many times in my life that I got to the point where I thought I'd never start again. I thought about that as I stepped up to speak to that audience, an audience that never dreamed they'd see someone like me standing up there as the highlight of their industry's evening. But there I was, and they were all ears.

"The creation of the Nike Fitness Innovation Award," I began, *"has provided the opportunity and the avenue to open our hearts and our doors and our programs to the inactive and the sedentary individuals in our society, thus breaking down long-held barriers and misconceptions."*

Right there, the crowd broke into applause. I couldn't believe it.

"Ladies and gentlemen," I continued, *"it's not about fat. It's about fit!"*

Another ovation. This was fantastic.

"*Fitness,*" I went on, "*is not about size. It's about life. Enhancing and lengthening the quality of our lives. To our students, our members, our friends, our loved ones — it's about providing the tools to accommodate everyone, regardless of size or fitness level. That's the goal and the design of my program.*

"*Take the intimidation out of participation,*" I told them. "*We can effectively bridge the gap between those who accept fitness into their lives and those who have felt excluded from the promise and the possibilities of fitness.*"

They were right with me, every soul in that ballroom. I could feel it, just the way I can feel that connection in the workout room, when everything's in sync, when you're linked to one another as if there's no separation between any of you, as if you're all one person, one unit. That's how powerfully I could feel the emotion in that room as I moved toward my final words.

"*I invite you to join me in our grandest venture,*" I said, as the whole audience rose to applaud. "*Getting people off the couch and into fitness.*"

Now they were all up, four thousand men and women, each representing hundreds of people who already enjoy the fruits of exercise and each capable of reaching out to thousands more who do not, all of them standing and cheering on this night for one of those thousands of men and women who know how it feels to be on the outside looking in. Cheering — I still can't believe it — for me, for my idea, my dream, my goal, which is to take fitness outside the boundaries of the fitness industry and make it available to everyone.

I will always be thankful for the "leg up" that was made

possible through the Nike Fitness Innovation Award. My message was heard that night, and I have no intention of ever letting it go unheard again.

"*In the name of fitness,*" I said, as the clapping continued and I tried not to cry, "*Let's just . . . do . . . it!*"

13

Doing It

I want to take you to "my place." I go there on a regular basis, and it's like no other place in the world. Sometimes I arrive in my place and the sun is shining on my face, my earphones playing my Kenny G. or some Earth, Wind and Fire, or maybe a little Hootie and the Blowfish. My heart is pumping, the air is clean and sweet, my muscles are working, my body moving, my feet pedaling away — not too fast, but a nice steady pace — on my twelve-speed bike, and I feel so alive. . . . I feel *electrified*!

I can stay in this place as long as I want to. Nothing can hurt me, nothing disturbs me. Whatever downside is going on in my life doesn't seem quite so down. Time slows to a soothing flow. I feel happy, and content, and at peace.

That's what exercise does for my brain and my body.

Or maybe it's a step class in a room filled with bodies of all shapes and sizes. The music sets a beat and we move and sweat together, our brains become clear and so do our bloodstreams, as if our veins and arteries were being swept clean to make way for those endorphins.

Those endorphins! Let me tell you, those happy little campers are two hundred times more powerful than morphine of the same dosage. No lie. That's a medical fact. A drug more powerful than anything anyone's ever grown in a field or created in a chemistry lab is chugging along right there in our bloodstreams every minute of the day! It's natural.

It's incredibly healthy, with no side effects but happiness and well-being. And it's yours for the taking, twenty-four hours a day.

Activity, exercise, is the key. That's what opens the door to those endorphins. That's what opens the door to my "place," something food never could do. Food for me was an instant gratification fix with nothing left after but a stew of guilt, emptiness, and sadness. Now it's different. Now, when I am stressed, do I take a short walk versus stuffing my face? Is there any doubt?

I'm not talking about running a marathon here — but we could! I'm not talking about a pedal-to-the-metal workout. I'm talking about simply moving, period. Moving to cope rather than eating to cope — or working yourself to death to cope, or sucking on a joint to cope, or draining a six-pack to cope — that's the first step. A healthy habit pushing aside something not so healthy. With exercise, with moving, I not only feel good during it, but I also feel the lingering thrill *after* it, which is something food never did for me. After the "eating thing" of the past, I always felt so much worse than I did before. It was only *during* the eating that I got any satisfaction at all, and that was so fleeting. Eating was an escape, a form of checking out. Exercise is about checking in! It lasts, it builds, it grows. It is, in a word, a lifestyle. It's not something I *do* so much as something I *am*. Taking my activity away from me now would be like taking *me* away from me. Don't even think about it.

This is my "place." It's sacred to me, as precious as anything in my world. Now I want you to think about *your* place. If you don't have one yet, write down what you would like your place to feel like if you did have one. What do you think you might have to do to get there? What would you like to do to get there?

You *can* do it. That is the essence of the message of my program. That is what I've learned through my own journey, and that is what I've shared with my hundreds and hundreds of students.

Believe it, and you can achieve it. Each of us has the ability to make our own magic. It's a gift of the soul. You have everything to gain and nothing to lose.

So let's start right now. You've gone where I have been. I've shared my guts and glory. Now it's time to make this all apply to *you*. I want you to own your own New Face of Fitness. Think of me as your one-on-one partner.

MOVING YOUR MIND

First off, you need to realize that there are so many choices for you when you begin to reshape and redirect your body — and your life — to true fitness. My goal is to take you

through some specific examples, then lay out the smorgas-
bord of choices and let you pick and choose as you begin to
make your own magic!

It's vital to remember that in order to really change,
we've got to work on ourselves from the inside out, to work
on ourselves not only physically, but mentally and emotionally as well. You may want to work on one behavior in
one area at a time; you may be up to working on two behaviors in two areas at the same time; maybe you'll feel
comfortable working on one thing in each of the three
areas. A warning: too much too soon may result in overload, which can lead to overwhelm.

Example: Betty decides this January first that she's not
only going on a diet, but she's going to quit smoking, she's
going to begin seeing a therapist weekly, and she's going to
join aerobics! WOW!

She finds dieting is so complex, with the measuring,
the weighing, the food portioning, the special food to
buy. . . .

Then she's got the therapist, whom she is squeezing
into her schedule, and the therapist needs her to open up
her entire life in painstaking, gut-wrenching detail, an
hour at a time, once, maybe twice, a week, which leaves
Betty emotionally wrung out, not to mention the nervous
glances she's giving her checking account. . . .

But she can't stop moving, because she's got to get to
her aerobics class, and being Betty, she's of course signed
up for the top-level "Aerobi-Kill-Ya" workout. . . .

And she has proudly not touched a cigarette in two
days.

On the third day she begins to shake. Overload is setting in. This whole jaunt is starting to overwhelm her body and brain. So much change, so fast. Betty finds she can't make it through her aerobics class. She's ready to kill for at least a puff of one smoke. She says to heck with the weighing and the food measuring and she goes straight for the Oreos. As for the therapist? Well, that was taking more out of her than putting anything in, and it didn't seem to be *going* anywhere. She could tell this guy her life story for the rest of her life, and there was no guarantee anything was going to change.

All or nothing. Now or never. That's the trap Betty was in, the human trap so familiar to so many of us. It got the best of Betty, and it will get the best of you, too, if you try taking on too much at once.

We are not going to do that anymore. I am not going to do it, and neither are you. It's that simple.

Grab a notebook, or staple a bunch of papers together. Go out and buy a nice journal if you like. Your book; your road map to your own magic.

First off, you have three parts that make up YOU. Your New Face of Fitness will include working on things in each of those three areas: the Physical, the Mental, and the Emotional (including the Spiritual). Make three columns on the page and write one of these headings above each column. Never forget that as you move your body, you will be moving your MIND. They go together. They work together. There is no separating the two, not on the path to true fitness.

Under the Mental heading, list at least ten things you like about yourself. Things such as:

I am fit.

I am a loving mother.

I am outgoing.

These are called affirmations. You know, most people can't say things like this about themselves. I don't care if you don't believe it, or if there are ten things you just wish you were. Write them down. Do it!

Now, the first thing you can do in the "retrain your brain" department is each morning, *every* morning (this only takes a few seconds), look into a mirror and recite to yourself the first affirmation on your list, such as "I am fit." Then finish this with "I love my body," and "My body is great." Stay with this affirmation, day after day, morning after morning, until you can say it without a cringe, without a smirk. In other words, say it until you mean it and believe it. It may take a few weeks. It may take a few months. But I guarantee you, if you do this, your perceptions about yourself and your body will change. And what are a few months when you're undoing a lifetime of treating yourself and your body without the care, compassion, and respect they deserve?

Understand that your body image has everything to do with your perceptions, that your self-esteem has nothing to do with your actual body shape and size. It's how you see it that creates the reality. I'm not talking about seeing yourself as something other than what you are. I'm talking about seeing yourself as you are, but shifting the filters and the angles and the *attitude* you've been laying on your body all your life, an attitude shaped and steered by others rather than by yourself. It's time to take control of yourself. It's time to live by your own rules. Not the fashion industry's rules. Not Madison Avenue's rules. Not your family's rules. Not your friends' rules. Not anyone else's rules but your own. No more negative thinking. It's time for some reality here.

Believe me, with that reality, with the creation of positive perceptions and a healthy body image, you'll find that doing things with that body, beginning to move it, to push it toward places it hasn't been in a long, long time — if ever — will be easier and more pleasurable, more rewarding, more fun than you'd ever imagined. Staying power will no longer be an issue. I guarantee it. This is what "retrain the brain" is all about — preparing that body to have healthy things done to it on an ongoing basis, as a lifestyle.

That's what your New Face of Fitness is — a *lifestyle*. It is not just exercise — exercise alone rarely includes the support, the rewards, and the behavior changes necessary to achieve a strong heart, body, and mind. It is certainly not a weight-loss program. Millions of people have lost millions of pounds through dieting and / or exercising and where has that gotten them? Where has that gotten *us*? Why do we continue as a society to careen in the direction of dissatisfaction and dis-ease when it comes to our bodies and our health?

Your personalized New Face of Fitness is your own place, an individualized recipe for health and wellness that works. It's not a quick fix, a gimmick, a new promise to change your life overnight, a cure-all. It's about loving yourself, and using that as fuel to take the unhealthy aspects of your life — be they physical, mental, or emotional — and effectively turn them in the direction of health.

Carefully. Progressively. Gradually. That's the way to incorporate exercise into your life in a meaningful way, to improve the cardiovascular and other body systems, along with muscle conditioning and toning, behavior modifications, self-esteem-building concepts. That's the way this program — this new face — works. That's the approach you need to take if you choose to launch your journey alone, and it's the approach we use at every New Face of Fitness site across the country, where I have created a fun, nonintimidating atmosphere, with instructors who as often as not are overweight themselves, who are works in progress themselves, just like my students, just like me, just like you.

Keep that in mind. We are all, always and forever, from the cradle to the grave, works in progress. That's what it means to be human. That's what it means to be alive.

Here are a list of reminders I'd like you to write in your notebook under the Mental heading. Call this list a Reality Check. Responding to each of these statements, considering whether it is true for you right now, and if it is not true, doing everything in your power to make it true, will be a powerful first step toward reshaping your life. Notice I didn't say anything about reshaping your *body*. Where the mind goes, where the attitude goes, where your approach to your life in general goes, your body will follow. Always keep that in mind.

Write the following twenty statements in your book, then consider each one carefully in terms of how you are living your life right now, and in terms of any changes or adjustments you might like to try making in your life.

1. My self-talk is primarily supportive and positive. I'm my own best friend!

2. I am able to separate my behaviors from who I am. I'm not "good" or "bad" because of what I eat or how much I exercise.

3. My feelings about myself are basically consistent with the way others perceive me.

4. I don't spend time comparing myself to others.

5. I accept every compliment I get with a smile and a thank you.

6. I like my beliefs and my interests and am willing to stand up for myself with no apologies.

7. I like the way I express myself when I move my body.

8. I make an investment in myself to feel attractive — flattering clothing, good haircut and makeup, quality food — no matter what I weigh.

9. I have made peace with my body — even if I'm not perfect.

10. My base of self-worth includes attributes other than physical attractiveness. I don't use the scale or my jeans size to determine my worth.

11. I set realistic goals based on what I really want rather than on what others think is best for me.

12. I continue to focus clearly on my goal — knowing that difficulties and delays cannot deter me from my vision.

13. I always keep in mind that each small step I accomplish brings me closer to my final goal.

14. I stay open to feeling my feelings to help guide me along in my journey.

15. I surround myself with the people in my life who share my "as if" reality.

16. I refuse to call myself the old negative names I had for myself (i.e., "gross," "disgusting" . . .).

17. I reinforce my new perceptions of myself by repeating them to myself at least five times a day (i.e., "I am strong," "I am graceful," "I am athletic").

18. I minimize the time I spend with people who are unwilling or unable to perceive me in a different way from the past.

19. I make sure my "as if" reality affects my behavior, my actions, the way I move, the way I think, the way I carry myself, and the way I interact with others.

20. My imagination is my strongest ally.

GETTING OUT OF THE GATE
Overcoming Exercise Resistance

> *"I know I'd feel better if I just got some exercise, but I can't seem to get motivated."*

*"If I could just lose a little weight first, it would be eas-
ier to start working out."*

"I don't like to sweat. It makes me feel gross."

"I'm too heavy."

"I'm too klutzy."

"I'm too embarrassed."

"Forget it. I don't have the time."

Do any of these statements sound familiar to you? Almost everyone knows that more activity would be good for
them, but so many of us can't seem to get motivated. We
really don't know how to begin. And we've got a million and
one excuses to fall back on.

Thousands of us actually start exercising but quit
pretty quickly, even when we find we're enjoying the activity. Thousands more of us say we hate exercise, period, and
don't even start. Then there are those of us who are interested, but put it off, telling ourselves we'll "get to it some
day."

Motivation is about more than just getting started. It's
about staying with it as well, and it's not a simple matter,
not for the tens of thousands of men and women who have
fallen prey to the variety of ways in which exercise is connected to and twisted by unhealthy features that should
actually have nothing to do with it.

Such as:

1. Exercise is so often associated with dieting, which has
   a 95 percent rate of failure. Most people will fail on

their diet and quit their exercise program as well. They then associate failure with one with failure with the other.

2. Exercise is too often used to change the body into a culturally accepted shape. For many women, quitting exercise is connected with a despair over society's sex role stereotyping, which encourages women to get in shape as a way to increase their personal value by becoming more sexually attractive. Men and women who try to change their body with exercise for this reason are too often disappointed and quit when they see that they are not approaching that ideal shape.

3. Exercise is too often used as an external measure of self-worth. In our culture, exercise is revered as something that supposedly reflects on a person's character, their inner strength, a testimony to their worth. Conversely, if you're *not* exercising, you're judged on those same terms, in a negative way.

4. Exercise is often used as a form of self-punishment, a response in a negative way to eating too much or not losing as much weight as we want, or simply gaining weight. We've been "bad" or "self-indulgent," so it's time to work out, to pay the debt.

5. Sexual abuse is sometimes connected in a deep way to exercise resistance. Moving the body can bring up body memories of early abuse. Exercise can actually trigger flashbacks of repressed abuse by restimulating a part of the body where trauma has been stored. Many victims of trauma stop physical activity either immedi-

ately after the abuse begins, at puberty, or at some point where they feel sexually or physically objectified.

It's vital to be aware of all these possibilities in terms of your physical, mental, and / or emotional response to activity. It's just as vital to shift the purpose from goals of weight loss, competition, or perfection to a focus on pleasure, nurturance, self-fulfillment, social and psychological benefits, energy boosts, and a sense of self-mastery. The decision to exercise needs to come from deep within. So many false starts with exercise occur because the person — man or woman — is doing it for externalized reasons, such as "I should do it for my health" or "I need to lose weight" or "My partner really wants me to."

The decision to exercise is about reconnecting with your body. Making a commitment to becoming more physical will have a deep impact on your internal experience. Changes in your *external* condition, in your body shape and size, are merely a side effect and have to be seen that way. If that external stuff becomes the focus, it will do nothing but damage to the whole process, and you'll be right back where you started.

The fact is that some inactive people who are considering exercise are not ready for it yet. Some self-examination is necessary before taking the first steps into actual activity. First and foremost, and from the beginning, this is about *movement*, about the joys and benefits sheer, simple movement can bring us if it's approached the right way.

It doesn't hurt to conduct a little personal survey before you even begin your own program of activity. Try the following couple of exercises:

1. Watch a group of children play for thirty minutes. Make careful observations and write them in your journal.

2. Play with a child where the child has freedom to move around. Pay attention to the details of how that child moves and feels. Also pay attention to how *you* move and feel. Enter those observations into your journal.

The joy of movement. That's the focus here. How many of us still experience as adults the unrestrained, unchecked, unlimited pleasure of simply moving our bodies that we enjoyed as children? How many of us even remember it? Reconnecting with that feeling is at the core of overcoming exercise resistance.

MOVING YOUR BODY

Most people don't realize how little physical activity is needed to be healthy, that it doesn't have to involve an exercise regimen or routine, that it can — and *should* — be an effortless part of day-to-day life, like bathing, or brushing your teeth.

The mainstream media with its barrage of hype and images, its go-for-the-burn, manic portrayal of exercise, virtually ignores the benefits of less intense, more enjoyable forms of physical activity. And the public — you, me, and Joe and Jill next door — wind up totally discouraged by these ultra-sleek creatures from another planet and so we just do nothing.

Check this out. A recent study found that health benefits begin for those who burn up as few as five hundred calories a week, and death rates decline by 20 percent. Five hundred calories a week. That's a fifteen-minute walk each day. Or two hours of bowling. Hey, my *grandmother* bowls. In other words, just getting up and off the couch, just standing up and walking around, just moving, period, is literally a healthy first step with direct results.

Take it easy. For most of us, exercise is best undertaken in a noncompetitive environment with activities that nurture self-esteem. The biggest mistake most people make is pushing too hard too soon. A slow and gentle start is so important. Initially, don't even think about goals or about "fitness." Think of pleasurable activities that can be done in the course of the day, as a natural part of your life, and preferably without structure. Things like hoeing a garden, digging and pulling weeds, maybe pushing a lawn mower, are a great first step toward incorporating a regular routine of movement into your life. Simple activities like these can increase the heart rate of a sedentary person by as much as 25 percent. That's a significant start.

Or try an occasional swim. Or forget the actual swimming — just bounce up and down in the pool.

Or dance.

Or bat a tennis ball back and forth with a friend (no keeping score!).

Or bat a tennis ball against a wall by yourself.

Or toss a Frisbee with a friend.

Walk the dog.

Walk yourself, with no goal of "exercise." Instead, pick some flowers along the way, with the goal of coming home with a nice fresh bouquet for the dining room table.

Take an extra trip around the mall before heading out to your car.

After a drive to the supermarket, carry all the groceries into the house rather than asking someone to help — go ahead, make an extra trip or two.

Rake leaves.

Shovel snow.

Make love.

And know that every bit of activity counts and adds up to better health, especially in the beginning. Don't expect improvement overnight. In fact, don't expect *anything*. Just do it. Pay attention to the sensations in your body, the slightest changes in body temperature, in skin moisture, in your breathing. These are all natural results of physical activity, and you know what? They're *gooooooooooood*. They might seem a little odd, even a little uncomfortable at first, but they're not unbearable, that's for certain, and the rewards, the way you'll feel after those initial sensations have passed, will make you want to go out and do it again. And again. And you'll be *enjoying* it, which is the essential ingredient here, the one that will keep you from quitting.

Another key to getting started and *staying* with an activity is to visualize the specifics of what you plan to do. Don't just tell yourself, "I'm going to start taking walks." Ask yourself where you are going to walk. When? Whom will you walk with? What will you wear? What will you do if it rains while you're walking? The same questions go for any activity you choose. If you plan to play ball with your child, ask yourself when, where, with what ball, for how long? These questions, as basic as they might seem, give a context, a frame of reference, a shape and a structure to the activity. They make the activity less open-ended, and therefore less easy to drop or drift away from.

The same affirmation exercise used in front of the mirror in the morning to shape your attitude about yourself can be applied to activity itself. Paying attention to your body sensations as you begin to move, take those sensations and turn them into positive statements to yourself, statements such as, "I feel my strength when I move." Or "I like myself and feel easy in my body when I do this." If and when your body shape begins to change, try not to say to yourself, "Hey, I've lost weight." Try instead to take that observation one step further, to looking specifically at how you feel, at how your body feels, with the changes that are taking place.

Avoid at all times talking about fat, about burning calories, about losing weight, or about appearance. Also avoid talking about exercise. None of these things are what matter most. What matters most is how your body and mind and soul feel.

THAT's what fitness is about, and that's what I mean when I talk about the New Face of Fitness: it's about fitness, not fatness. Thin people aren't always fit, and heavy people are not always unfit. You've heard of Isadora Duncan, the fabled dancer? She was a big woman, as was two hundred-pound Virginia Zucci, a world-class Russian ballerina, famous for her pirouettes. Lynne Cox, the world record holder for swimming the English Channel — that includes men's times as well as women's — is five six and weighs 180 pounds, with 33 percent body fat.

As you get ready to start moving, take a close look at what might have been holding you back in the past. Answer the following ten questions, looking closely at any "Yes" answers and asking yourself what you might need to do to change those answers to a "No," so you can begin taking true fitness into your own hands.

Hint: turn each statement into a positive affirmation, and you'll be on your way. Example: if your answer to number 1 below is "Yes," try writing down the phrase "I will move to feel good" or "I will move to sleep better." Put that phrase on the fridge, write it in your journal, say it to yourself in front of the mirror, and that will shift the "Yes" answer to a "No." It won't happen overnight. It's like everything else, you're going to begin with a lot of doubt and disbelief and eye-rolling at yourself, but stay with it, give it time, and you will believe it. And you will achieve it:

1. I almost always exercise to burn calories.

2. I see exercise as a necessary evil.

3. I use exercise to try to change my body into a culturally accepted shape.

4. I get disappointed with exercise when my body doesn't come close to that ideal shape.

5. I (or my doctor, family, etc.) use exercise as a measure of self-worth.

6. I tend to rebel when told I should exercise.

7. I use exercise as a punishment when goals such as a limit on food intake or weight loss are not accomplished.

8. I view my body as bad and self-indulgent.

9. I despise my body being warm or sweaty.

10. I have been sexually abused and have not dealt with this through professional counseling.

THIS WONDROUS MACHINE

As you begin moving your body and you begin tuning in to how it feels, noticing how it responds to activity — how your skin feels, how you're breathing, what your muscles are doing, how your joints are reacting, how you feel after the activity as well as how you feel during it — it's important to understand where those sensations are coming from, sensations you might never have felt before in your life. It's important to understand the basics of body mechanics. You don't need a Ph.D. in anatomy or physiology to understand the fundamental principles that guide the beat of your heart and the rate of your breathing. And understanding those principles will help immensely as you begin shaping your New Face of Fitness.

Let's start with the heart. Two words are all you need to know: stroke volume. That's the term for how much blood your heart is able to pump with each beat. A weak heart pumps less blood per beat than a strong heart, which means it has to work harder to push that precious fluid through the body, which means it will wear out quicker and be more prone to damage and disease.

Take me as I was six years ago. I weighed well over three hundred pounds, and my blood pressure was through the ceiling. Why? Because my poor weak little heart was beating a mile a minute every minute of the day just to do the job of keeping me alive. My resting heart rate at that time was 75 b.p.m.'s (beats per minute). Today my resting heart rate is down to 65. At first glance you might say, So what? Well, take a second and think about it. That's 10 pumps per minute that my stronger, more efficient heart is not having to work at. That's 600 pumps per hour — 14,400 pumps per day — 100,800 pumps per week — 403,200 pumps per month — more than 4 million pumps per year.

Tell me that's not going to add up to some extra years of life. What else in the world can give you *more life*? Money can't buy it. Influence can't lure it. Success can't bring it, and neither can power. There's only one key that unlocks that magic door, and that's fitness. And the beautiful thing is that this magic is there for everyone. It doesn't belong to the rich or the powerful. It doesn't care about age, or gender, or race. All you have to be is human, and it's yours for the having.

Okay, so we can see how the heart is helped when the body begins moving. Let's see, what's next? What else besides our pounding hearts do we immediately notice when we begin moving our bodies? That's right — our breathing. This is where the term *aerobics* comes in. It means, literally, *with oxygen.*

Take a look at that phrase. *With* oxygen. Not without. *With!* For the longest time I connected the term *aerobics* with the breathless leaping, pounding, bounding acrobatics shown on TV workout programs. Out of breath. Panting. Gasping. That was aerobics to me. And that's where I — and anyone else with that vision of this kind of activity — was wrong.

Aerobic activity has nothing to do with thong-clad jumping to the moon. If anything, recent research shows quite the opposite. High-intensity activity does not necessarily have to be high-*impact* activity. It's a high-intensity workout we're after, and you can get that through low-impact exercise.

For example: you may get much more benefit out of a steady twenty-minute walk than you can trying to run the same distance in ten minutes. Even if you finish that run in one piece, you haven't necessarily done your body any good. And you may well have done it harm if you're pushing it too hard. This depends, of course, on where you're at when you start! Ten minutes at a faster pace after three to six months could be great. The bottom line is there is no "Always" or "Never." We are all different! We are all unique!

Healthy, beneficial, efficient aerobic activity involves finding your own pace, your comfort zone, if you will, and working your body within that zone. Stay tuned to your heartbeat and your breathing and you can't go wrong. And you will keep going. That's the name of the game. Go. Move. Keep it up. And enjoy it. Exercise is not about suffering. It's about enjoyment. Incredible, huh? Who would have thought it?

Okay, now let's talk about the "F word." Fat. The human body is made up of lots of stuff, but let's look at it right now in terms of two categories. Fat, and everything else. That "everything else" is called lean body mass. The fat is called — you guessed it — fat mass. When you do aerobic activity, you are not only strengthening your heart and increasing the efficient flow of oxygen into your system, but you are also building muscle mass. You can't help it. Strength means muscles. Muscles mean strength. I'm not talking about the outsized biceps and calves and pecs you see all greased up and shining on stage in those bodybuilding contests. I'm talking about real-life muscle, muscle for use, not for show, muscle for life.

From the minute you begin moving your body, you will be building muscle, though you may not see it. But it's happening. And the fact is that it takes more calories to maintain muscles in the body than to store fat, and muscles burn more calories than fat (even at rest). You can probably see where this is leading, but stay with me.

When I first heard years ago that exercise built muscle, which helped burn fat, I thought that meant the muscle would literally replace the fat. I pictured myself turning from a three-hundred-pound couch potato into a three-hundred-pound muscle-bound freak. What a choice! Every pound of fat would change into a pound of muscle. That's what I thought.

Well, of course that's not the way it works, but what did I know? What do any of us know about things we haven't looked at? Well, when I began actually looking at this matter of muscle — when I began seriously studying physiology on my way to becoming a professional instructor and personal trainer — I learned quickly that muscle is muscle and fat is fat and each develops in its own way. As you begin exercising, and you are working aerobically, and your heart is beating more efficiently, and you are burning calories, your muscles begin to develop and get stronger and redirect those calories long before your fat begins to disappear.

Revelation! You'll *be* it before you can see it. Those muscles will be changing inside you long before the fat you see on the outside begins slipping away. Add to this the fact that muscle is denser and thus heavier than fat, and it's easy to see why so many of us become confused and even discouraged when we first begin a regular routine of exercise.

Take Sally. She could be any of us. Sally starts exercising and dieting and decides to jump on the scale every week (maybe every day) to see how she's doing. About six weeks into her new routine, which she is following religiously, she has actually gained a pound. Her clothes are looser on her body, but the number on the scale hasn't dropped! Sally is perplexed. And she is dismayed. And she is discouraged. And more likely than not, she chucks the whole thing, says to heck with it, reopens the food floodgates and winds up back where she started and even worse, because now it will be that much harder for her to believe in the benefits of exercise. After all, she gave it a go and where did it get her?

If Sally had only known, she was well on her way. Unfortunately she was done in by what she didn't know. *And she was hoodwinked by that mesmerizing monster that lurks in bathrooms and locker rooms throughout this country* — the scale.

Get rid of that thing. Throw it out. You don't need it. You don't need to know how much you weigh. What does it matter how much you weigh? To whom does it matter? It's a number. That's all, and so what?

It's time to put a New Face on this matter of body measurements, on gauging how fit we are. What matters is how your body feels and what it can do. Period. How your body looks is a byproduct, something that will take care of itself. I'm not saying it doesn't matter. Of course it matters. But it should not, and it cannot matter most. When it stops mattering most, when our focus shifts from the outside to the inside, from form to function, that is when change will truly take place. Real change. Healthy change. Happy change.

Have you ever tried looking at something in a completely dark room and found that if you look straight at it, it's hard to see, but oddly enough, if you look slightly away from it, you can actually see it better? It's the same way with so many things in our lives. Sometimes the best way to see something clearly is to stop looking at it directly. Sometimes a shift of focus, looking somewhere else for the answer, is the key to getting unstuck.

That's what the New Face of Fitness is about. A shift of focus. Getting unstuck.

TIME OUT

As you embark on your own fitness journey, as you begin to get up and get moving, as you start exercising in whatever way, shape, or form you choose, be it bowling or tossing a boomerang, walking or weeding, working out in your living room or actually joining a program like mine, you need to be aware of the limitations of your body, especially if you are among the majority of American men and women who live with special conditions ranging from arthritis to diabetes to high blood pressure to, yes, being overweight.

None of those conditions mean you can't be fit. Fitness is for *everyone.* Some people simply have a few more things to consider and take into account than others as they begin exercising and strengthening their bodies.

If you are one of these people — and most of us are — here are some specifics to keep in mind, some adjustments to make as you begin working out. These adjustments are known in the fitness industry as "modifications."

High Blood Pressure

- No overhead activity with the arms raised.

- Keep to low-impact activity with pulse rate no higher than 140 beats per minute (walking, low-impact aerobics, swimming or water-walking in a pool, all at a "walk-and-talk" pace).

- Non-weight-bearing movements are preferred.

Overweight

- Low-impact, fat-burning movements are preferred (basic Step-Touch aerobic movements, knee lifts, heel-ups, side-out abductions — movements that work the large leg muscles, front and back, inside and outside — again at a heart rate no higher than 140 beats per minute).

- Frequency of activity: 4 to 6 times per week; for de-conditioned people, starting with 2 to 3 workouts per week and working up to 4 to 6 is recommended.

- Train at a heart rate of approximately 140 b.p.m.

- Non-weight-bearing movements are preferred.

- Emphasize duration of activity rather than intensity.

Arthritis, Knee/Joint Soreness, Surgeries

- Range of motion is the focus.

- Avoid extreme extension and flexion.

- Those with arthritis should expect to feel pain during activity; they need to distinguish between "normal" pain and "beyond" pain, using the Two-Hour Pain Rule:

Two-Hour Pain Rule: If you are still experiencing pain beyond what is normal for you two hours after you have stopped exercising or later, you should adjust your activity accordingly. (Let's say you're using two-pound weights to do bicep curls, and later that day you notice your wrists are killing you, that there's more than normal pain; the next time you do bicep curls, just let the muscle do the work, without using any weights at all, or cut back to one-pound weights; remember, let your body signals be your guide.)

- Avoid overloading joints that are sore or swollen.

- Avoid high-impact, weight-bearing movement.

- Avoid jarring movements.

- Avoid side-angle movements.

Diabetics

- Blood glucose should be monitored more frequently when beginning exercising.

- Exercise consistently with regard to time of day, intensity, duration, and frequency of activity.

- For insulin users, inject insulin into areas that are not used heavily during exercise (abdomen or arms preferred).

- Eat complex carbohydrates

- Snack 20 to 30 minutes before working out, especially if blood sugar is low.

- Avoid exercise when diabetes is not controlled.

- Keep in mind that exercise can have positive effects
  on the body, actually lowering the insulin requirement.

This last point, the fact that exercise can actually alter
the body's limitations, is true not only of people with diabetes, but of people with any of the limitations listed
above. Aerobic exercise that is consistent over a long term
not only may extend your life, it will *change* it.

Exercise can literally be *healing*. Believe it. It's true.

FINDING YOUR GROOVE

So now you're ready to find your groove. You're getting up
daily and you're looking in the mirror and moving your mind.
I love my body, and my body is great. It takes a whole three seconds.

Next you've decided that walking is going to be the best
place for you to start in terms of an activity. Before you step
out that door, however, you need to take care of getting medical clearance from your doctor. Every athlete who tries out
for an amateur or professional sports team undergoes a
physical before the first day of practice. It's necessary. It's required. It makes sense. Well, the same goes for me. And the
same goes for you. This is not an option. This is not a sug-
gestion. This is a *must*.

When you go to the doctor, tell him or her how far
you'd like to walk, how fast, and how frequently. Listen to
what he or she tells you in terms of setting up safe guide-

lines and modifications for your physical activity. And when you venture out onto the sidewalk, or the track, or climb onto a bicycle, or buckle up a pair of Rollerblades — whatever your choice of activity is — *listen to your body!*

Say you choose to walk at a talkable pace for five or ten minutes. Evaluate how you feel at the end of that time. Are you panting? Does your side hurt? Do you feel light-headed? If you feel good, try walking for five to ten more minutes. Now, if you're a little huffy and puffy after that, stay at that level for a while. Don't try to push it. If you're feeling good and sweaty but you're not in any actual pain, then you're in the right range. Your body will let you know. And as you get stronger, you'll be able to go longer.

Frequency, duration, and intensity. Those are the three magic words when it comes to planning your actual physical activity.

Frequency: how often will you do it?

Duration: for how long?

Intensity: how hard, or at what pace?

Depending on the level and combination of these three components with whatever activity you choose, you can raise your cardiorespiratory fitness level (that percentage of heart rate described back in Chapter 7, the one recommended by the American College of Sports Medicine) by anywhere from 5 to 30 percent. Your cardiorespiratory level, which is a fancy term for oxygen uptake — the amount of oxygen you're able to take into your body and efficiently absorb — is one of the most basic barometers of fitness. And according to the ACSM, the fact is that the 30 percent figure, the high end of improvement in oxygen uptake from exercise, occurs among "*individuals with low ini-*

tial levels of fitness, cardiac patients, and those exhibiting large losses of body weight."

That's straight from the 1995 edition of the ACSM's guidelines. In other words, if you are inactive, out of shape, or "deconditioned," as the experts put it, the changes in your body's response to a regimen of healthy exercise and nutrition will be more dramatic and more immediate than the changes felt by people who are already active to one degree or another.

In other words, you've got more to gain in the beginning — more improvement to enjoy, more changes to be awed by — than people who are already active. That's one more reason to get up and get moving!

But how often?

How far?

How hard?

It's tough to know the answers to these questions if you're just starting out. In fact, you can't know them. But there are some things you do know. You — along with your doctor — have already taken a good look at your body and its limitations, whatever those might be. Your activity could be any of the following:

Solo

Bike riding

Walking

Rollerblading

Jogging

Swimming

Skating (ice or roller)

Group

Step aerobics

Low-impact aerobics

Circuit training

Interval training

Lateral motion training (slide)

Team

Baseball/softball

Volleyball

Basketball

Soccer

Hockey (street, field, or ice)

Alternative/Extreme

Mountain biking

Rock climbing

Kayaking

Mind/Consciousness

Yoga

Meditation

Stress/relaxation exercises

Whichever activity you might choose, either from this list or elsewhere, you certainly need to familiarize yourself with the basics in terms of equipment, if there is any, and in terms of necessary skills, if there are any. Armed with that fundamental knowledge — of your body and of your activity — the only way to find your most beneficial level in terms of frequency, duration, and intensity is to wade in and get wet. Explore your body. Explore your self. Explore your activity.

Start . . . doing . . . it.

But do it wisely. Nice and easy. If it's too easy, push it a little bit. But don't hurry.

According to the ACSM, improvements in cardiorespiratory endurance, along with caloric benefits, can be *"best met in sessions lasting 20 to 30 minutes,"* not counting time spent warming up and cooling down. If that seems like too much, fine, says the ACSM. *"For severely deconditioned individuals,"* state the guidelines, *"multiple sessions of short duration (about 10 minutes) may be necessary."*

The point is, start slowly, then push on out according to what your body tells you it is able to do. You've got the rest of your life to find your own limits, whatever they might be, whatever your needs and desires might be, whether you want to change your level of fitness or, once you reach a certain point, simply maintain it. No need to go too far too fast and risk possible injury.

Like yours truly.

About a year and a half ago I found out that my right knee, my patella, had come a degree or two off its tracking. It had been bothering me for some time, that sharp, stabbing type of pain in a joint that lets you know there's more wrong there than just soreness or aching. I went to my doctor, and what he deduced was that way back when I got started with this whole fitness thing, that first year at Gigi's, I was so big and my muscles were so pitifully weak, that my frame could not support the strain of suddenly moving all this weight around.

Did I know then how important strength training is as an ingredient in overall fitness? No, I did not. Back then, and for the longest time, it was believed that strength training shouldn't be done by people who are deconditioned, or overweight, or elderly, the reason being if you don't know what you're doing with weights and equipment, you'll hurt yourself. Which is true.

But continuing research has shown that strength training builds muscle density and mass *and* helps decrease body fat composition. When you build muscle mass, you burn calories better *and* you decrease your risk of injury because you're building a stronger musculature to support the movement of your body in your chosen activity.

If I were starting over, along with my beginning aerobics activities I would work on strengthening my trunk and stabilizing my major joints through basic strength training exercises.

The same goes for you. Whatever your choice of aerobic activity, I would couple that activity with *strength training*. And let me emphasize that strength training does not necessarily mean weight training! You don't need weights to work on building your muscles. You can do a complete, efficient, and effective strength training session without lifting a soup can. Resistance exercises, where you push against a wall, or another person, or against yourself (you've heard the term *isometrics*, meaning one set of muscles is tensed by pressing against another set of muscles or against another object?) can be done in the comfort and convenience of your own home.

I can't overemphasize the value of strength or resistance training in tandem with aerobic activity. Besides the direct benefits of increasing the strength and mass of your muscles, the physiological benefits of this kind of training include increases in bone mass and in the strength of body tissue, especially, says the ACSM, among *"middle-age and older adults, and, in particular, post-menopausal women who rapidly lose bone mineral density."*

Other benefits of strength or resistance training?

- improvements in cardiorespiratory fitness

- reductions in body fat

- modest reductions in blood pressure

- improved glucose tolerance

Again, how much? For how long?

Well, most experts in muscular strength and endurance recommend the following guidelines for resistance training, as listed by the ACSM:

Intensity

• Perform one set of 8 to 10 exercises that train all the major muscle groups (e.g., gluteals, quadriceps, hamstrings, pectorals, latissimus dorsi, deltoids, and abdominals). Each set should involve 8 to 12 repetitions to the point of volitional fatigue.

Frequency

• Resistance training should be performed at least twice a week, with at least 48 hours of rest between sessions.

Duration

• Sessions lasting longer than 60 minutes may have a detrimental effect on exercise adherence. Adherence to these guidelines should permit individuals to complete total body resistance training sessions within 20 to 30 minutes.

Okay, we've got the aerobic activity down, we've got the muscle-building covered. Before we move on, there's one more thing we need to do with our bodies, and it's just as important as strength or aerobic conditioning. I'm talking about *flexibility*, particularly in your lower back and rear-of-the-thigh areas. Neglecting those two spots can open you up to the risk of chronic lower-back pain — the bane of so many weekend-only athletes. Everyone needs to stretch as part of their physical activity routine, but it's especially vital among the deconditioned and the elderly. In fact, studies have shown that a well-rounded program of stretching can actually counteract the usual decline in flexibility among elderly men and women.

Again, according to the ACSM, here are the guidelines for stretching exercises:

- Always precede stretching exercises with some type of warm-up activity to increase circulation and internal body temperature.

- Stretch smoothly and never bounce.

- Do not stretch a joint beyond its pain-free range of motion.

- Gradually ease into a stretch, and hold it only as long as it feels comfortable (10 to 30 seconds).

Intensity

- Exercises should incorporate slow movement, followed by a static stretch that is sustained for 10 to 30 seconds.

- Exercises should be prescribed for every major joint (hip, back, shoulder, knee, upper trunk, and neck regions) in the body.

- Three to five repetitions of each exercise should be performed.

- The degree of stretch achieved should not cause pain, but rather mild tension.

Frequency

- Stretching exercises should be performed at least three times a week (preferably daily) and should be included as an integral part of the warm-up and cool-down routine.

- Devoting an entire exercise session to flexibility may be particularly appropriate for deconditioned older adults who are beginning an exercise program.

Duration

- The stretching phase of an exercise session should last approximately 15 to 30 minutes.

One last thing I'd like to suggest about the list of sports and activities included in the middle of this section: explore it. Try out as many of these activities as your body can safely handle. Your brain will hold you back more than your body. Softball? Bowling? *Hockey?* You might not be able to even imagine yourself trying most of these activities. Well, *imagine* it. Then try it. And you just might be amazed at what you discover in terms of a whole new dimension to your life. Don't be afraid of failing, because failure isn't even in the picture anymore. Remember? Trying is success. The mere fact that you're *trying* on those Rollerblades, or you're *trying out* a four-person game of beach volleyball, or you're *trying* to stretch those thigh muscles and break a sweat in that 10 A.M. step aerobics class — the mere fact that you're getting out there and exploring these activities, enjoying the spirit of adventure, *trying* to take your body and your health into places they've never been, means that you . . . are . . . SUCCEEDING.

Remember, we're opening our brains and bodies to possibilities. Choices. Different strokes for different folks. That's what life is all about, and that's what you'll see and believe with your New Face of Fitness:

That life is not about limits; it's about possibilities.

HABITS
Retraining Your Body and Your Brain

Water.

That's where I started, the first habit I focused on when I began taking my fitness into my own hands back in 1989. I had my positive pumps — my affirmations — going each morning, I was into the activity end of things at Gigi's, and now it was time to turn to the food-and-nutrition end of things. I'd learned how the process of hydration works, how important it is, and how it's often linked to what we perceive as hunger. But I'd never paid attention to drinking water before then. Are you kidding me? Why would I bother with a glass of water when there was a world of food to enjoy?

I started with a glass per meal, and let me tell you, it was a drag. I used every trick in the book to fake myself out. I'd buy Evian (my very favorite), pour it into a nice crystal glass with ice cubes (made with Evian), add a twist of lemon, and pretend I was in a chic restaurant where the menu was written in French. The experts call this "imaging," and it works.

Once I had the one glass per meal going, I started adding glasses at other times of the day. I made sure I had sixteen to twenty ounces with me during my aerobics class, which I drank before, during, and after class. I would write down the total ounces I drank per day, and I would reward myself at the end of each week, selecting from a list of rewards I drew up for myself: a hot bubble bath; shopping with a friend; a bike ride; listening to my music; a massage; going to see a good movie; buying myself something frivolous; getting a pocket book for a friend and myself; a manicure; a pedicure; lunch with a friend. Those were the sorts of things I had on my list. Think of the things you'd like on yours, and write them down. And use it. And don't be amazed when you find yourself drinking 100 ounces of water a day, the way I did after my first year on this routine — the way I still do today.

That was my first habit. Others followed, one at a time. Keep that in mind. *One at a time!* It's easy to get excited with a taste of success. You can get carried away trying to change too many things at once and wind up overwhelmed and laid out with that old O-ring syndrome. Nice and easy. Steady as we go.

Once I had my water habit going, the next habit I turned to was not cleaning my plate. *Not* cleaning my plate. Let me tell you, that took some time. It was pretty ridiculous in the beginning. I mean, I'd leave one pea at the edge of my dish, or a couple of crumbs in the corner of what had been my cake plate. Still, that was more than I'd leave before. That was a beginning. That was success! And one pea became two, and three, and after a while, if I had a serving of meat, potatoes, and veggies, I would leave a

little bit of meat, a couple of pieces of potatoes, and a few
of those veggies, and call it quits. That's not to say I didn't
start off with a *huge* helping. I know it might sound comi-
cal, this bigger-than-big blonde chick in a restaurant heaping her plate a mile high with food and then leaving this
teeny little bit at the end. But that's exactly what I did. I
had no timetable. No beating myself up for meeting or not
meeting this deadline or that.

Nice and easy.

Back to that mountain of food I began with. It would
be so easy, so tempting, to try tackling that sucker right off
the bat. But I'd learned, oh how I'd learned, that that way
lies certain failure. This was a new game plan. I would
eventually get at that mountain, but not head-on, and not
directly.

My next habit was an inner thing — paying attention
to the difference between being stuffed and being satisfied.
That took some doing. We all know what stuffed feels like.
Turkey days. Thanksgiving. Christmas. The cornucopia of
the holidays. That's what stuffed feels like, and some of us
have been in a place where that feeling is a way of life, day
in and day out, not just at holidays and times of indul-
gence, but at every meal. That's what compulsion is like,
where the thing you're doing is in charge of you rather than
vice versa, where you're continuing to put food into your
body far past the point of pleasure, even beyond the point
of discomfort. When I began pulling back and paying attention to how my body felt as I ate, I was gradually able to
stop stuffing myself and gear back to being simply full.
Then I geared back a bit more to being simply satisfied. It
took months — it took years — but little by little I was able

to do it (I'm *still* doing awareness checks on myself in that department).

All the time I worked on one habit at a time, I kept working out with my activities, and I kept starting my mornings with those positive pumps, and when I noticed that that one habit was leveling out, that it had become just that — a habit, something routine that I no longer had to *try* to do — then I moved on to another one. Eating breakfast, for example, something I never used to do. Now it's at least a piece of fruit or yogurt, wheat toast, or a bagel.

I suggest that you make a Fitness Habits Sheet to help you track your progress with each "habit" you choose to tackle. Remember, awareness is a central ingredient of commitment — using a chart to track your habits is a great boost for awareness.

FUEL

Eating.

For far too many of us, for far too long, what we put into our bodies has become the end-all and the be-all of our lives. We obsess over what we eat, how much we eat, when we eat, where we eat, *whether* we should eat. We shape our moments around what we put into our mouths, making it larger and more significant than anything else in our lives. We crave food, we hate food. We chase food, we hide from food. We devise elaborate strategies to allow ourselves to wallow in what we eat. We devise desperate strategies to enable ourselves to avoid it. We take the simple stuff of sustenance — our daily bread — and we turn it into both an altar at which we worship and a cross on which we crucify ourselves.

It's time now to change all that. It's time now to redefine our relationship with food — just as we need to redefine our relationship with whatever other unhealthy coping mechanisms might be damaging our lives — and that's what it is, a *relationship*. Like our husbands or lovers, like our children and friends, like everyone and everything that is essential in our lives, for better and for worse, we must learn to establish a healthy relationship with food. We can't live without it, just as we can't live without the people we love. We need it, just as we need them. But it's not good for us, it's not *healthy* for us, to give it power over us, just as it's not healthy to give another person power over us, no matter how much we might love them. A healthy relationship with anyone or anything is about balance and perspective. It's about giving everything in our lives its proper weight, importance, shape, and size, not making it larger and more significant than it is and not making it smaller and less important than it should be.

This is the way we need to deal with food. We need to understand it, just as we need to understand our loved ones. We need to know what it can and cannot give us, just as we need to know what our husbands and children and friends can and cannot give us. We cannot — or should not — try to squeeze out of it something that is not there, something that is actually found elsewhere, just as we should not expect or demand the people around us to fill needs in us that are meant to be filled by something else. We can destroy a relationship when we strain and twist it by putting expectations, demands, and disappointments where they don't belong. It's that way with people. And it's that way with food.

Think about it. When something we eat is labeled as bad, it becomes something to be avoided. Well, the first thing that happens when you purposely avoid something is that you tend to think about it more than ever. The more you try to stay away from it, the more important it becomes.

Bad or good. Healthy or unhealthy. By setting up these labels, we're setting up a trap. We're pushing food away from its proper and natural place in our lives and turning it into an object of judgment. By shifting our thoughts and feelings about food from a neutral into a judging position, we lose touch with our feelings about food, just as we lose touch with our feelings about our bodies when we turn activity and exercise into mere means to weigh or look a certain size or shape. Just as understanding, getting in touch with, and listening to the sensations of our bodies can guide us to a happy, harmonious, *healthy* place, so does getting in touch with, learning about, and listening to our experiences of the things we eat.

Our body can show us the way to eat if we let it, if we pay attention to it. I mean really pay attention, unclouded by the buzz and static of our thoughts and hangups and judgments and needs that don't — or shouldn't — have anything to do with food. In a way, it's not unlike a form of meditation. Unlike what most people think, meditation is not about checking out of this world. It's not about sitting in a lotus position, closing your eyes, and going away to some blissful place, escaping from the world. Quite the contrary, meditation is about checking *in*. It's about clearing the mind of the chatter and noise and thoughts and ideas that get between us and the experience of the moment so that we can experience the moment. Clearly, fully, without the filters of our thoughts. It's about being right here, right now.

This is what we need to do with food. Tune in to it. Pay attention to it. The smell of it. The taste as it enters your mouth. How it feels as it is swallowed. How it feels as it makes its way into the stomach and begins to be digested. The resulting energy level it gives you. The clarity — or cloudiness — you feel when you're done. How long the sense of satiety or fullness lasts.

In other words, rather than obsessing about the food itself, pull back and pay attention to yourself as well, to how your body responds to and is affected by food throughout the entire process of both eating and digestion.

Trust your body. Pull away the layers of expectations, good or bad. Pull away the screen of judgment. Let food be just what it naturally is. When we moralize about it, when we label it bad or good, then we begin labeling ourselves with those same terms and the downward spiral begins. No longer are we in charge of our feelings about ourselves. We're handing those feelings over to food, giving it the power to make us feel good or bad about ourselves.

There is no question that we need to understand nutrition. We need to know about food, about the sources of protein, the benefits of fiber, the need for as well as the dangers of fat. But we need to be constantly alert as we begin studying food not to become obsessed with it and to fall into the good / bad trap. That leads to distance and distrust rather than joy and satisfaction. And joy and satisfaction are what we're looking for in food, just as we're looking for it in every aspect of our lives — true, healthy joy and satisfaction.

Here are a few guidelines to help stay on track in terms of our relationship with food:

1. ***Avoid terms that have moral overtones or convey value judgments.***

   Because "food guilt" is already rampant in our culture, it's important to avoid using judgmental terms when thinking about food, eating, or weight. For example, instead of saying, "I'm eating too much fat, and that's bad for me," try saying, "I know that people who eat a lot of fat often feel sluggish. Is that happening to me?" Consider the difference between the following two statements:

   "My blood glucose is high because I cheated."

   "I notice my blood glucose goes high when I eat ice cream after dinner."

   Look. Listen. Feel. But don't judge.

2. ***View food in context with the other areas of your life.***

   Don't pound yourself with notions of this or that eating habit or food choice being bad or good. Pull back and pay attention to the effect this or that eating habit or food choice has on your body and your activities before and after eating. No food is good or bad in and of itself. Broccoli is not inherently "good." Chocolate syrup is not inherently "bad." It's what these things do to our bodies, to our energy levels, to the way our lives are lived that matter, and those things are not "good" or "bad" either. Happy or not happy, yes. Satisfying or not satisfying, okay. But not "good" or "bad." There are too many layers to those terms, they go too deep, and they almost always get us off track.

3. *Appreciate the social context of eating.*

Imagine you're playing cards with your son. He's eating tortilla chips, you're munching on carrots — but would much rather have the chips. How "healthy" are those carrots in this situation? Although you're trying to connect with your son, although you're there, in that moment, to enjoy the card game, your focus has slipped from the game to the food. The game has become secondary. It has become something you happen to be doing while you're eating. Try shifting the focus back to the game. *That's* the context.

4. *Use needs as the basis for evaluating the fuel you put into your body.*

Think of going to a service station to fill up your car's gas tank. You're faced with some choices when you get to the pumps. If you're driving a car with a diesel engine, you're going to look for the diesel pump. You know that non-diesel fuel could ruin your engine. For a gasoline engine, you have several choices. The owner's manual suggests which specific grade of fuel is best for your car. Or maybe you learned by trial and error, by trying one grade of fuel, noticing your car "pinging" as you drove it, and trying a different grade the next time. Adjusting. Seeing how the fuel affects the engine and the ride. Listening to your car's feedback and responding appropriately. The fuel itself is not "good" or "bad." Some fuel works for some cars; other fuel works for other cars. Finding the right "fuel" for your body — and that's exactly what food is — involves the same process of listening to your own engine's feedback to find the fuel that gives you the best "ride."

5. *It's not what you're eating; it's what's eating you.*

When we talk about food, it's vitally important to keep in mind that we're not just talking about what we eat; we're talking about our *relationship* to what we eat, our response to what we eat. In other words, we're talking about behaviors. We're talking about *habits*. We're talking about actions and attitudes about food that are shaped by experiences and needs and feelings that have nothing to do with food. Knowing that, exploring those needs and feelings while initiating and developing a happy, healthy routine of activity, we can begin altering our food-related actions and responses — those habits — one at a time.

Okay, with the proper attitude, both about ourselves and about food, we're ready for information, so here are the basics of healthy nutrition, the dietary guidelines established by none other than the U.S. Department of

Agriculture and the Department of Health and Human Services. Keep this as a reference, and you can't go wrong. These guidelines are the best, most current advice from nutrition experts.

- *Eat a variety of foods*

  Eating a variety of foods — not a few highly fortified foods or supplements — is the best way to get the energy, protein, vitamins, minerals, and fiber you need.

  No single food can supply all the nutrients in the amounts you need. For example, milk supplies calcium but little iron; meat supplies iron but little calcium. To have a nutritious diet, you must eat a variety of foods.

  Any food that supplies calories and nutrients can be part of a nutritious diet. It's the content of the total diet over a day or more that counts.

  Use the Food Guide Pyramid to help you eat better every day:

  ## The Food Guide Pyramid
  A Guide to Daily Food Choices

  Fats, Oils & Sweets
  Use sparingly

  Milk, Yogurt & Cheese Group
  2–3 servings

  Meat, Poultry, Fish, Dry Beans, Eggs & Nuts Group
  2–3 servings

Vegetable Group
3–5 servings

Fruit Group
2–4 servings

Bread, Cereal, Rice & Pasta Group
6–11 servings

Start with breads, cereals, rice, and pasta. Go heavy on the vegetables and fruits. Don't ignore the items toward the top of the pyramid, but go easier on them. They're as necessary as the things on the bottom, but in smaller amounts. Remember, no one food group is more important than another. For good health, you need them all.

- *Choose a diet low in fat, saturated fat, and cholesterol*

Many Americans have diets high in fat, saturated fat, and cholesterol. These diets are linked to increased risk for heart disease, obesity, and certain types of cancer. Here are healthy goals for fat and saturated fat; keep in mind that these goals apply to the diet over several days, not to a single meal or food:

Total Fat

Your goal for fat depends on your calorie needs. An amount that provides 30 percent or less of calories is suggested. The chart below shows the upper limit on the grams of fat per day that corresponds to various daily calorie intakes:

Calories	Total Fat per Day	Saturated Fat per Day
1600	53 grams or less	Less than 18 grams
2200	73 grams or less	Less than 24 grams
2800	93 grams or less	Less than 31 grams

Saturated Fat

An amount that provides less than 10 percent of calories is suggested. All fats contain both saturated and unsaturated fat (fatty acids). The fats in animal products are the main sources of saturated fat in most diets, with tropical oils (coconut, palm kernel, and palm oils) and hydrogenated fats providing smaller amounts.

Cholesterol

Animal products are the sources of all dietary cholesterol.

Food tips to reduce fat, saturated fat, and cholesterol:

- Use fats and oils sparingly in cooking.

- Use small amounts of salad dressings and spreads such as butter, margarine, and mayonnaise. Try reduced or non-fat substitutes.

- Choose lean cuts of meat and trim visible fat.

- Take skin off poultry.

- Have cooked dry beans and peas instead of meat occasionally.

- Moderate the use of egg yolks and organ meats.

- Choose skim or low-fat milk and non-fat or low-fat yogurt and cheese most of the time.

- Check labels on foods to see how much fat and saturated fat are in a serving.

- **Choose a diet with plenty of vegetables, fruits, and grain products**

  Eat more vegetables, including dry beans and peas; fruits; breads, cereals, pasta, and rice. A varied diet that emphasizes these foods supplies important vitamins and minerals, fiber, and complex carbohydrates and is generally lower in fat.

  It's better to get fiber from foods that contain fiber naturally rather than from supplements. Some of the benefit from a high-fiber diet may be from the food that provides the fiber, not from the fiber alone.

- **Use sugars only in moderation**

  Sugars and many foods that contain them in large amounts supply calories but are limited in nutrients. Sugar comes in many forms, such as table sugar (sucrose), brown sugar, honey, syrup, corn sweetener, molasses, glucose (dextrose), fructose, maltose, and lactose.

  Use sugars in moderation — sparingly if your caloric needs are low. Diets high in sugars have not been shown to cause diabetes.

Both sugars and starches — which break down into sugars — can contribute to tooth decay. Avoid excessive snacking, brush your teeth with a fluoride toothpaste, and floss regularly to help prevent tooth decay.

- **Low-fat eating out**

  It's easier to control how much fat you eat when you or a family member is doing the cooking. But what about when you're eating out? You can usually find tasty, low-fat alternatives on the menu. And if you can't, ASK! Ask for sauces and dressings on the side, steamed dishes, and foods that are grilled or baked without added butter or oil. Here are some suggestions for low-fat choices:

  Fast Food

  Fast food can mean "fat" food. Stay away from french fries, breading, cheese, and special sauce. Some good choices are:

  - Single broiled hamburger with mustard, tomato, lettuce, and pickles
  - Broiled, grilled, or baked chicken, fish, lean beef, or lean pork
  - Salad (avoid eggs, bacon bits, croutons, and too much dressing)
  - Turkey or lean ham sandwich (with mustard instead of mayonnaise)

Italian

Italian food can be healthy if you avoid cream sauces and too much cheese or meat. Some good choices:

- Pasta with marinara or tomato clam sauce
- Pizza with vegetable topping (not olives) and half the cheese
- Pasta or potato gnocchi in tomato sauce
- Minestrone soup

Mexican

Avoid fried or refried foods, guacamole, sour cream, and too much cheese. Some good choices:

- Tostadas, enchiladas, or fajitas
- Steamed tortillas
- Whole beans and rice
- Baked cornmeal tamales
- Soft (not fried) tacos

Asian

Avoid breaded and deep-fried dishes. Some good choices:

- Steamed vegetables and rice
- Steamed vegetarian pot-stickers or dumplings

- Chicken, fish, or lean beef or pork steamed, cooked in broth, or broiled
- Hot-and-sour or wonton soup

Supermarketing Tips

Deli Counter

- Sliced roast beef, turkey, and lean ham are low-fat choices.
- Pressed meats, lean ham, and Canadian bacon are low-fat but high in sodium.
- Turkey and chicken franks do not always have less fat than beef franks; some are merely smaller. Check the nutrition label for sodium and fat content.
- To limit fat, try salads made without creamy dressings.
- If processed lunch meats are used, select those marked 95 percent fat-free.

Dairy Case

- Try plain, low-fat yogurt as a mayonnaise or sour cream substitute in chilled dishes.
- Look for part-skim mozzarella, scarmorze and string cheese; part-skim or low-fat ricotta; and "light" and reduced-calorie cheeses that contain less than 5 grams of fat per ounce.

- Milk, buttermilk, cottage cheese, and yogurt that are low-fat and have less than 200 calories per serving are good nutritional choices.

- A little sharp cheese has more flavor and less fat than a large amount of milder cheese.

Bread and Cereal Shelves

- Look for cereal with at least 2 grams of fiber, 8 grams or less of sugar, and 2 grams or less of fat per serving.

- Compare portion sizes and calories on cereal labels; servings range from ¼ to 1¼ cups.

- Look for the words "whole wheat" or "whole grain" at the beginning of the ingredient listing. "Wheat flour" is nutritionally equal to white flour.

- If selecting white breads, choose enriched ones.

Canned Food Aisles

- Choose 100 percent pure fruit juices instead of fruit "drinks" or "punches."

- Dry coffee creamers are mostly saturated fat and sugar. Evaporated skim, low-fat, or whole milk are better choices.

- The edible bones of canned salmon and sardines provide calcium.

- Canned beans, peas, corn, and vegetables are quick and easy sources of vitamins, minerals, and fiber.

- Check sodium levels of canned foods if your sodium level is restricted.

Packaged Products

- Limit products with palm, palm kernel, or coconut oil high on their ingredient list.

- Thick, unsalted pretzels are lower in fat and sodium than most other packaged snacks.

- Graham crackers, animal crackers, ginger snaps, and fig bars have less sugar than most other cookies.

- Most microwave popcorns are high in fat and sodium. Make your own in an air popper or with a limited amount of oil and butter-flavored substitute or cooking spray.

- Rice and pasta mixes are high in sodium; use only half of the seasoning packet.

Fats, Oils, and Dressings

- Soft, tub margarines and spreads are made with unsaturated oils.

- Regular butter and margarine have 100 calories per tablespoon; spreadables have 80 calories per tablespoon; whipped varieties have 70 calories per tablespoon.

- Some "light" oils are light only in color and flavor, not in fat or calories.

- "Light" mayonnaise has about half the calories of regular mayonnaise.

Meat Counter

- Select lean, well-trimmed cuts: flank steak, round steak, or roasts, sirloin or tenderloin, loin pork chops, 85 percent lean ground beef.

- Meat graded "Select" has less fat than "Choice" or "Prime" grades.

- Lean beef, pork, and lamb are not much higher in dietary cholesterol than poultry or fish, but they have more saturated fat.

- Beef liver is very high in iron, zinc, and many vitamins, but it is also high in dietary cholesterol.

- Limit high-fat meats such as ribs, corned beef, sausage, and bacon.

Fresh Fish and Poultry Sections

- Half of chicken's calories are in the skin. Buy skinless parts or remove skin of cooked poultry before eating.

- Fish from deep waters have heart-healthy omega-3 fatty acids: salmon, tuna, mackerel, sea trout, bluefish, herring, bonito, pompano.

- Fresh ground turkey is a low-fat substitute for ground beef.

- Most chicken and turkey nuggets, patties, and rolls are made with ground skin and have a lot of salt.

Frozen Food Cases

- Purchase frozen fish and poultry without breading to limit fat and sodium.

- Look for frozen dinners with less than 15 grams of fat, 400 calories, and 800 milligrams of sodium.

- Frozen concentrates are often the least expensive form of fruit juice.

- Ice milk and low-fat frozen yogurt have less fat than ice cream.

- Plain frozen vegetables have less fat and salt than those in sauces.

- Frozen juice and fruit bars with no added sugar or cream are good choices.

- Portion-packed frozen desserts help curb the tendency to eat large helpings.

All right, there's the nitty-gritty on nutrition. Finally, I strongly recommend an immensely useful tool to use in conjunction with your work on habits. It's called a food journal. It's amazing what the simple process of paying attention to what you eat can do to your eating habits. It's amazing what we aren't aware of until we stop and look at it. The food journal is a way of stopping and looking.

And remember — I can't emphasize this enough — the whole process of dealing with food is *not* to make it your adversary. Enjoying food is one of the many delightful pleasures of being a human being, of being alive. If our relationship with food has become skewed, let's look at tweaking that relationship a little bit, bringing food back into our lives as a pleasurable, healthy, *fun* experience. Awareness is the first step to health in any form, be it exercise or eating. So here, in terms of eating, is one last checklist to help you become aware of your own behaviors and which ones you might like to pay attention to. Answer each of these questions as brutally honestly as you can, and keep answering them as you make your way along the path of true fitness — they, along with the other "reality checklists" in this chapter, will help keep you on track:

1. I have kept a food journal to record my food, feelings, and situations and to understand why I might be eating more than my body needs.

2. I usually keep a food journal whenever I'm having a hard time with my food and weight.

3. I am in tune with my physical hunger and begin most of my meals hungry.

4. I know how to stop eating when I am physically satisfied and usually do so with no problem.

5. I am able to eat almost any food without beating myself up or feeling guilty.

6. I almost always take action to handle feelings and situations that trigger me to eat by:

   • identifying the feeling/situation.

   • making a choice between feeling uncomfortable or addressing the issue.

   • reaching out for appropriate support from family and friends.

   • engaging in counseling if I see my problems are not changing.

7. I am not stuck at just "wanting"; I am willing to do whatever it takes. (This refers to changing your *relationship* with food, as well as setting limits, saying no, and so forth.)

8. My attitude toward my body is "If you can't be with the one you love, love the one you're with."

9. I practice numerous nurturing behaviors to fill myself so that I don't need to turn to food.

10. I usually know what my needs are and how to get them met by setting limits and communicating directly.

11. I assert myself and rarely have to resort to yelling, arguing, or feeling frustrated with others around me.

12. I acknowledge that making an effort to lose weight without meeting these reality checks will always be counterproductive.

FINALLY

The last thing I'd like to say about these various stages of incorporating activity and healthy eating habits into your life is that while it's possible to take this journey alone, it is incredibly rewarding — not to mention helpful — to join others who are taking the same trip. If you can surround yourself with friends and loved ones — actually, almost anyone who joins you on this journey will become a loved one, I guarantee it — you'll find that the entire experience will become enriching beyond your wildest dreams. That's one of the fundamental foundations of my New Face of Fitness program, that we're all in this together and we can feed off one another's energy. I've seen the magic happen in studio after studio, in city after city, all across this country.

If you want to become a part of that magic, by all means come on in. You can call or fax the New Face of Fitness to find the center nearest to you or to be put on our newsletter mailing list (see page 223).

In any case, whether you join my program, whether you join your neighbors and friends, or whether you go solo, I want to wish you the best and welcome you to *your* place. If it feels half as good to you as mine does to me, you'll be in heaven — heaven right here on earth.

And don't we all deserve that!

Epilogue

It's the start of another summer, and I'm looking out the back door of our new house — our rented house — in Panama City, Florida, watching my boys splash in the pool and trying to figure out how to free up some time for my afternoon bike ride.

That's right. Panama City. The Coast Guard transferred us again in the spring of '96, and now we're back beside the good old Gulf of Mexico, with Keith spending his days on search-and-rescue patrols and the occasional hunt for Caribbean contraband, and me setting up yet another household, getting the kids enrolled at yet another school, meeting yet another circle of new friends and neighbors.

We left in May, Keith and the kids and I packed into our Chevy truck and pointed down the interstate. We made a few stops on the way — in Wheeling, West Virginia, and Greenville, South Carolina, and Columbus, Georgia — all part of the tour I'd been making since January, launching New Face of Fitness classes at YWCAs from coast to coast.

What a whirlwind! In the wake of that Nike award back in '94, things just took off in terms of travel and exposure. The people at Nike were eager to do whatever they could to help make New Face of Fitness available to the millions of Americans who might respond to it if they knew about it. When the YWCA came on board, offering to include the program at their operations in thirty cities across the country, with more to follow if those went well, we were on our way.

I mean that literally. Over the course of six months, beginning in January of '96, I flew from city to city, lugging my bags through airport terminals and in and out of rental cars and taxicabs, making my home in hotel rooms, taping my affirmations to the walls and mirrors of every Marriott and Ramada Inn between Portland, Oregon, and Trenton, New Jersey . . . and leaving those little notes behind to pump up the spirits of the staff coming through to get those rooms ready for the next customer.

The pace was crazy. Most days I'd fly into a city, hop in a rental car, and go straight to the YWCA site, never mind checking into the hotel. There was no time to check into the hotel. Some sites were set up as if the *Pope* was coming to town — huge banners, balloons, and a crowd of staff and members there to welcome me as if I were royalty or something. Other places, I'd get there and have to help set up the chairs. Did I mind? Are you kidding? Whatever it takes, I'll do. Whatever it takes.

I arrived at every one of those cities charged up for a full day — or two, or even three in some cases — of being *on!* The morning meet-and-greet with members and instructors — always at least several dozen, often more than a hundred — followed by a motivational address, then a workout. After that, some media interviews — newspapers, radio, TV. Then lunch, followed by afternoon sessions that as likely as not would last into the evening. Sometimes I wouldn't check into my hotel room until after ten at night. By the time I settled in and was ready to sleep, it would be one, and the alarm would be set for five because I had to get to the airport first thing in the morning to catch a flight to the next city.

There were days during the first couple of months of this that I thought I was going to die. I went from doing twenty workouts a week on Governors Island to riding in airplanes and sitting in rental cars and rushing to hotel rooms, and even though I was teaching demonstration classes, I did not feel right. I did not feel good. The fact was, I was feeling *fat!* I hadn't gained any weight, but I was feeling fat. It got to the point where I had to have a serious sit-down with myself, review where I was and what I was doing, and realize that I'd been ignoring one of the basic messages I'd been preaching to people since this whole thing got started, which is that life never sits still, everything shifts, everything changes, and if you think you're going to come up with one plan that will take care of everything in your life now and forever, forget about it.

After a little soul-searching and realizing it was okay — no, make that *necessary* — to carve out some time and space each day for myself, no matter where I was or what I was doing, after reassessing my on-the-run, on-the-road eating habits and putting a little more care into my menu selections — more salads and fruit plates (dressing on the side), more fish and broiled chicken, more bagels and yogurt, and, of course and always, more WATER — and after making sure I at least walked the halls of the hotel for a half-hour if I didn't do a full-fledged workout that day, I was back on track.

That mental feeling of fatness went away. I haven't lost any weight in the past year, but I'm happy to tell you I haven't gained any either, which is a great achievement given my regimen during that time. I just finished going out and buying three bathing suits for this summer, and they're the same sizes they were last year — 14's, 16's, and 18's. Isn't that lovely? You bet it is.

Constant adjustment. It's a part of life. And you know what else is a part of life? Pain. That's right. I get a dozen or more letters a week from women and men across the country telling me how their New Face of Fitness has changed their lives, and let me tell you, the joy in those letters is matched by the pain so many of them — so many of *us* — have had to deal with in the past and still struggle with today. I'm not talking just about physical pain, though there's plenty of that. We all have our emotional baggage, and some people's is heavier than others'. I got a letter just last month from a woman in Lincoln, Nebraska, who told me of the "disappointment, disgrace, and accusations" she had feared before she gathered the courage to attend a workshop I held at the YWCA there. Her letter went on:

> *I am an adult survivor of child molestation. I am*
> *convinced my self-esteem breakdown is a direct result*
> *of my childhood. In combination with this circum-*

stance, my weight is extreme. I eat as a coping mecha-
nism. I have searched a long time for a place I could go
and be accepted for who I am. I'm willing to give this a
try if it will give me an opportunity to deal with my
past while overcoming my struggle with my self-image
and bringing closure to my pain.

I don't know that there is ever such a thing as bringing closure to that kind of pain. I don't know that that kind of pain ever does go away. This too shall pass? I don't think so. Getting rid of our pain is not the issue. How we *cope* with that pain is the issue. Finding a new plan. Finding new tools. That's the key. The pain doesn't change; we do!

I still get sad. I still feel lonely. I'm always going to have that void, that place that was carved out inside me such a long, long time ago. It will never be filled. But isn't it wonderful and freeing to now realize that I have these brand-new healthy habits, these lifestyle tools to reach for each and every day? Isn't it fantastic that I don't have to sit there and think about how I've *got* to exercise today, or I *should* get that workout this afternoon, that I don't have to talk myself into anything anymore because it's mechanical now, it's a *habit*? If I go two days without activity, my body is screaming PLEASE TAKE ME OUT AND MAKE ME SWEAT!

I can never give you the words to describe how wonderful that is, considering how I used to sit on the couch and just be miserable. The mere thought of getting off that couch was impossible, much less doing it. I am by no means a small person today, but I don't even think twice about putting on my bathing suit and walking out with my friends and jumping in the pool. I'm no Daryl Hannah, and you know what? It doesn't matter. It's how I feel about *me* that enables me to put my suit on with joy and to relish the sensation of soaking in that pool.

Speaking of how I feel about me, it's important to point out that I am more aware than ever of how I feel about other people. I remind myself all the time to resist the temptation to judge, to leap to conclusions, to forget that there's more to everyone than meets the eye. I spent a couple of days in Cleveland during my tour, and one afternoon an instructor named Bonnie handed me a letter but asked me not to open it till later. This was the cutest girl in the world, the perfect Barbie-doll figure, the perfect personality, just the perfect person — the kind of person I would have felt ashamed to even be in the same room with not long ago. And now she was asking to shake my hand not once but twice, so she could take that home to her husband.

Or the woman in Lincoln, Nebraska, who was there all morning and all afternoon, too, hauling a rack out of a back room so we could hang our giveaway T-shirts on it, her husband right there with her, the two of them taking part in the workout, seated up front for the motivational address, sharing lunch, even lending a hand with the cleanup that evening. Her name was Vicki. I gave her a big hug when everything was wrapping up — we all give each other hugs at the end of the day — and she walked with me out to my car, just to say good-bye and tell me again how wonderful the day had been.

As I climbed in to start the engine, I watched Vicki make her way to her own car and noticed for the first time, because I think it was the first time all day she had used it, that she was tapping her way across the parking lot with a cane.

Vicki was blind. She told me so in a letter I received about a week after I got home:

> *I have been losing my vision since Nov. 1995. It took over one year to diagnose the problem. I felt suicidal at times. This past January I decided "New Face" would be just the thing to take my mind off my troubles.*
>
> *I started with my doctor, who suggested I see the HMO nutritionist/therapist. She advised me this would not be a good time to start a program, as my life was in "crisis." I was given Prozac, for depression, and a drug for anxiety.*
>
> *Against all advice, I chose "New Face." My decision came through prayer.*
>
> *I've loved the program from the start. My trainers are terrific! Tonight I received an award for losing 6½ inches. But my greatest loss is my depression.*
>
> *After three months my vision has improved. The chemical injections I receive for my disease are dispersed and absorbed more effectively. My endorphins are pumping and I have more sound sleep.*
>
> *I am an image consultant and job resource counselor, Dee. My career depended on change. You've saved me.*
>
> *Thank you.*

I had no idea.

Do any of us really have any idea what's actually there when we look at someone and judge them? I do it. You do it. We all do it. We're at the bus stop or the doctor's office or wherever, killing time, and what do we do? We check each other out. We classify. We make conclusions. We judge. Oh, she's rich. That one's a snob. That one's a slob.

Someone takes a look at me, well, Gee, she's got on Nikes, she's got on all that fitness stuff, and she's *fat!* Wonder what she's doing with that stuff on? Is she trying to look like she's fit or what? I mean, she can't possibly be fit. Not at that size. At that size, she's got to be lazy, no good, poor, and she probably doesn't make her bed!

See the craziness in that? Because the fact is we don't know where that person came from or what they're dealing with at that very moment. When we start picking others out and discarding them, we forget what it feels like to be left out ourselves. Don't tell me you've never felt left out. Don't tell me you've never felt like a geek. Don't tell me you've never been in a situation where you felt totally confused, completely at a loss, in way over your head, and you didn't have a plan, and you didn't have an answer.

Well, you know what? If you can recall those feelings, chances are you won't be so quick to judge. It doesn't matter whether you're a medal-winning Olympic athlete or you're looking at one. It doesn't matter whether you're an eight-hundred-pound nightmare or you're looking at one. If you can remember one time, one situation where you really felt confused, isolated, left out, then you've found that common link that connects us all, the core of that place called compassion, the bond that ties us all together as human beings.

We're people, period, and that's more than enough to make us each worthy of love, especially from ourselves.

We've each got a heart, a heart hungry for connection and caring.

I feed mine every morning, when I wake up and look into the eyes of my loved ones, the family I now have with my boys and my husband.

I feed it every time I look in the mirror and see a woman I truly respect, understand, and embrace, someone I care about and care for every waking minute of the day.

I feed it when I meet and re-meet the members of my New Face of Fitness family all across the country, the women and men who write and call me and whom I write and call back, all of us sharing this incredible journey on which we've joined hands.

My heart, neglected and aching for so long, is fed to bursting these days, both with love and with fitness. And the fact is it's about time to feed it right now. We haven't been in Panama City long — I've still got boxes to unpack — but I've already discovered a killer twelve-mile bike loop along the bay not far from our house. It's unbelievably gorgeous. And it's a great workout.

Let's see, the boys have been invited over to a friend's to play. . . . Keith won't be back home for another couple of hours. . . . It's another to-die-for Florida afternoon, and my twelve-speed is pumped and ready to go.

Following is a list of individuals and resources specializing in or supplying information about fitness, training, nutrition, eating disorders, and obesity:

Dee Hakala
New Face of Fitness
P.O. Box 15668
Panama City, FL 32405
904-914-2466 (telephone)
904-913-8203 (fax)
On-line: Dee VVV at aol.com

Adrienne Ressler, M.A., C.S.W.
Director of Clinical Outreach
Renfrew Center
7700 Renfrew Lane
Coconut Creek, FL 33073
305-698-9222 (telephone)
800-332-8415
305-698-9007 (fax)

> *Adrienne is the director of clinical outreach for the Renfrew Center, a women's center specializing in the treatment of eating disorders, depression, and abuse issues.*

Erin Bohner, M.A.

809 Rosehill Ave.

Durham, NC 27705

914-416-0663 (telephone/fax)

> *Erin is a professional counselor specializing in working with addictive behavior.*

Eleanor Pella, R.D.

500 Camp Gettysburg Rd.

Gettysburg, PA 17325

> *Eleanor is the registered dietitian on staff for the New Face of Fitness.*

American Council for Exercise

5820 Oberlin Dr.

Suite 102

San Diego, CA 92121-3787

619-535-8227 (telephone)

619-535-1778 (fax)

YWCA of the U.S.A.

Dr. Alpha Alexander

726 Broadway

New York, NY 10003-9595

212-614-2700 (telephone)

212-677-9716 (fax)

American College of Sports Medicine

401 W. Michigan St.

Indianapolis, IN 46202-3233

317-637-9200 (telephone)

317-634-7817 (fax)

www: http://www.acsm.org/sportsmed

Certification Resource Center: 800-486-5643

International Association of Fitness Professionals (IDEA)

6190 Cornerstone Court East

Suite 204

San Diego, CA 92121

619-535-8979 (telephone)

619-535-8234 (fax)

800-999-4332

Nike Run-Walk Information

Dept. RLH

One Bowerman Dr.

Beaverton, OR 97005-6453

Acknowledgments

I'm sitting here thinking about whom I should dedicate this book to, all the incredible people I want to thank. To my grandma, Joan Gardner, a writer and poet. To my family, for surviving as best we could. To my husband, Keith, for "hanging," and to my sons, Zachary and Jeremy, for reminding me how precious life is. To God for allowing me this phenomenal opportunity called life, with its trials and tribulations, its lessons of learning, of pain and growth and huge amounts of happiness and sheer joy and thrill, and, above all, with the acceptance of self and learning to love me, too.

I want to thank Gigi Teeter and all the wonderful aerobic animals in Lake Charles — friends, colleagues, Mona and Carol and the whole limousine gang — for keeping the faith. Thanks as well to everyone who helped make Governors Island aerobics a reality and sweated with me there. Go Julie! Go Gail!

As a fitness professional, the help and assistance I received from IDEA, ACE, ACSM, AFAA, and the Renfrew Center has been invaluable. My special thanks to Adrienne Ressler and Karin Kratina.

I have learned the true meaning of empowerment from the YWCA of the U.S.A., where Alpha and all my "thirty little children" continue the mission. Thank you. My thanks also to the selection committee for the 1994 Nike Fitness Innovation Award. Without Nike's support, all this would have taken much longer.

Thanks to Eleanor and Elizabeth, the "E" gals. To Leslie Borasi, my continued gratitude.

My gratitude also to Catherine Crawford, David Black, and Michael D'Orso for "getting it." And to Beth Davey and Katie Long for "getting it — out there!"

My lifeblood is my "inner core circle." Words will never do justice to my feelings of gratitude to the following people: Paula Laird, Catherine Dupuis, Colleen Garvey, Erin Bohner, Roxie Greene, Scott Evans — your unconditional acceptance and support sustain me.

My thanks to Kristina Tallman for "steering the swan" in me and "bringing out the warrior" as well. You are the best!

Thanks to Ellen Langley for the gift.

To you, my reader, I thank you for reading this book and empowering yourself.

And finally, I thank "my dear sweet souls" — Susan Fox, Deli Parker, Myrna and Willie, Susan Clements, Charlie Spelts, and all the wonderful members and staff of our New Face of Fitness family, which grows larger every day.

This book is for us all, and I love you all for sharing with me and allowing me to be part of your life.